JUST 8 MINUTES A DAY TO
NO MORE WRINKLES

Looking great at any age depends on having beautiful skin. With this fabulous beauty expert's guide, you will discover how to keep your face, neck and entire body in top condition without surgery, without dangerous chemical treatment, without costly cosmetics. This is the same, instantly effective program of creative skin recipes, tips, and exercises offered in Constance Schrader's famous beauty seminars. Safe for all skin types, tones, and ages, this easy, inexpensive, 8-minute-a-day program brings you the radiant new complexion you've always dreamed of having.

CONSTANCE SCHRADER is a well-known skin-care expert whose corporate and continuing education seminars have achieved fantastic results for thousands of women and men of all ages. Her consumer and beauty articles appear regularly in *Working Mother* and other magazines. She has written five books on health and skin care, including *Youthlift* and *15 Minute a Day Facelift.*

NO MORE WRINKLES

And 500 Other Foolproof Tips for Younger, Healthier Skin

CONSTANCE SCHRADER

Introduction by George Serban, M.D.

Illustrations by Cathy Christy O'Connor

A PLUME BOOK

NEW AMERICAN LIBRARY

NEW YORK AND SCARBOROUGH, ONTARIO

NAL BOOKS ARE AVAILABLE AT QUANTITY DISCOUNTS
WHEN USED TO PROMOTE PRODUCTS OR SERVICES.
FOR INFORMATION PLEASE WRITE TO PREMIUM MARKETING DIVISION,
NEW AMERICAN LIBRARY, 1633 BROADWAY, NEW YORK, NEW YORK 10019

LIBRARY OF CONGRESS CATALOGING IN PUBLICATION DATA:
Schrader, Constance, 1933–
    No more wrinkles.
        1. Skin—Care and hygiene.   2. Skin—Wrinkles.
3. Beauty, Personal.   I. Title.
RL87.S35   1985   646.7′ 26   84-18621
ISBN 0-452-25609-7

PLUME TRADEMARK REG. U.S. PAT. OFF. AND FOREIGN COUNTRIES
REG. TRADEMARK—MARCA REGISTRADA
HECHO EN HARRISONBURG, VA., U.S.A.

SIGNET, SIGNET CLASSIC, MENTOR, PLUME, MERIDIAN
and NAL BOOKS are published *in the United States* by
New American Library, 1633 Broadway, New York, New York 10019,
in Canada by The New American Library of Canada Limited,
81 Mack Avenue, Scarborough, Ontario M1L 1M8

Designed by Kathryn Parise

First Printing, January, 1985

1 2 3 4 5 6 7 8 9

PRINTED IN THE UNITED STATES OF AMERICA

Contents

Preface

My skin seminars have reached almost 2000 people in the last few years. The information that I originally prepared was directed at wrinkle-fighting, but much of the class time was spent answering questions about texture, color, tone, and general loss of elasticity in skin. Everyone wanted a program that would make them look younger, fresher, softer—fast. It was because of demand for this sort of program that I developed the "Younger Skin in 20 Days" regime. It was tested by students in the seminars and modified, retested, and remodified. What we were looking for was a program that would fulfill eight criteria:

- It must bring immediate results.
- It must take no more than a few minutes a day. This was especially important to busy working women.
- It must be flexible enough to accommodate skin changes brought on by changing seasons, life-styles, and age.
- It must be simple and uncomplicated; easy to perform when groggy in the morning or exhausted at night.
- It must be inexpensive.
- It must work on all skin types, tones, and areas.
- It must bring lasting, beneficial results.
- It must be natural and inoffensive, with no negative side effects.

Everyone wants new skin—it's smooth, supple and younger-looking, with none of the blemishes and scars that inevitably flaw skin with time. There are several ways to achieve new skin: one way is deep-peeling, a very dramatic procedure done in a doctor's office. Another way is the natural renewal, achieved very slowly and mildly as your own skin grows and sheds every few weeks.

There are other methods, less radical than chemical peeling and faster than natural skin-renewal, however, that can give you new, younger-looking skin. One of the best ways I have found is what I call "Sugabrasion," which uses sugar to encourage the shedding of old skin. The Sugabrasion program fulfills all criteria for a workable program: It's easy, inexpensive, fast, and effective. And it is suitable for all skin types and men or women of any age.

The program is based on natural products: sugar, oil, water, and lemon juice or other natural acid. But before using these products to rejuvenate and protect your skin, you should know why they work, how they work, and how to control their use. You can be your own skin-care expert and change your program to suit your skin's natural fluctuations if you have an understanding of how your skin works. *No More Wrinkles* will give you all the information you need to put together a personalized skin-care program, a regimen that will give you newer, younger-looking skin.

So start now. You don't need expensive creams or salon treatments. All you need is the desire to have newer, softer, smoother skin instantly and naturally.

C. S.

Acknowledgments

I would like to thank *Network for Learning, Westwinds,* the *Watchung Community Center* and other sponsors for my seminars, and the hundreds of beautiful and delightful students I've had. Your questions and encouragement are greatly appreciated.

I would also like to thank Dr. George Serban, a wise and witty physician who has been very generous with his ideas and time; my husband Ernst who is also my best friend; Jean Brown who is the best listener in the world; and Agnes Birnbaum. Special thanks to my editors and the production department of New American Library.

SPECIAL NOTE

The reader should use personal judgment in using any of the programs described in this book, and in applying any of the natural beauty treatments. Each person's skin has individual sensitivities, and what works for some skin may have negative effects on others. Any adverse reactions, including muscular, physiological, or allergic reactions, as well as irritation and discomfort should be taken into account, and those activities or formulas should be avoided. Of course, no miracles from any beauty care—organic, muscular, or otherwise—should be expected or can be guaranteed.

Introduction

Throughout history, beauty has been a valuable and much sought after commodity, and never has a healthy, attractive appearance been more important than it is today. The cosmetics industry is now a multibillion-dollar business. And when cosmetology, the science of creating or enhancing beauty, seems to need a helping hand, plastic surgery stands ready to supplement its efforts.

Plastic surgeons attempt to reshape the body by correcting real and sometimes imagined defects in an individual's face, nose, breasts, or buttocks. The function such operations fulfill is social and psychological, and the price is sometimes exorbitant.

Usually plastic surgery is concerned with specific defects, whereas cosmetology deals with the general look of a person, from skin care to makeup. The efforts of cosmetologists and plastic surgeons or dermatologists do overlap somewhat in the area of skin care, however, particularly in the use of facial abrasion. Cosmetologists normally handle the minor problems, attempting to apply the principles of clinical medicine on a small scale. Unfortunately, what is medically right and wrong in skin care has not been definitively proven, which opens up the possibility of conflict between specialists and between cosmetologists and their clients.

The potential for confusion about skin care is aggravated by exaggerated claims for cosmetic products that promise terrific results but cannot deliver them. So great is the anxiety of people to achieve or maintain beauty that many continue to believe in the efficacy of various products and esoteric skin manipulations even after favorable results have failed to materialize. Others switch from product to product or specialist to specialist in an unending quest to look good. Especially for many women past forty, keeping the skin and body looking young and beautiful is no easy task, and many will turn to any cosmetic procedure that offers even a vague hope of success. The discrepancy between the modest results achieved by cosmetology in improving facial condition and the exaggerated claims for its benefits is large. Some skin treatments are little better than magic rituals—only the incantations are missing. Other procedures have good if not astounding results and contribute to the psychological well-being of the client.

In *No More Wrinkles,* Constance Schrader brings some much-needed clarity and direction to the field of skin care. On the basis of the latest scientific knowledge, she separates as much as possible fact from fiction—treatments for the maintenance of the skin which have real value from those that do not.

In addition, her book introduces new and creative methods for skin rejuvenation which aid in maintaining the youthfulness of the skin by removal of old skin cells through a process of sanding called Sugabrasion. This method accelerates the removal of dry, dead skin cells, leaving the skin looking younger. Another important component of Schrader's skin-care philosophy is a set of facial exercises which she calls "stimuslap," a form of mild massage intended to improve the skin's blood supply in the muscles beneath the skin, which has been recognized to be a vital addition to a good complexion.

No More Wrinkles is a valuable guide for skin care.

—George Serban, M. D.

JUST 8 MINUTES A DAY TO
NO MORE WRINKLES

Looking great at any age depends on having beautiful skin. With this fabulous beauty expert's guide, you will discover how to keep your face, neck and entire body in top condition without surgery, without dangerous chemical treatment, without costly cosmetics. This is the same, instantly effective program of creative skin recipes, tips, and exercises offered in Constance Schrader's famous beauty seminars. Safe for all skin types, tones, and ages, this easy, inexpensive, 8-minute-a-day program brings you the radiant new complexion you've always dreamed of having.

CONSTANCE SCHRADER is a well-known skin-care expert whose corporate and continuing education seminars have achieved fantastic results for thousands of women and men of all ages. Her consumer and beauty articles appear regularly in *Working Mother* and other magazines. She has written five books on health and skin care, including *Youthlift* and *15 Minute a Day Facelift.*

1

Are You Younger Than Your Skin?

Find Your Skin Time

Babies are usually born with healthy, smooth, flawless skin. But with the onset of puberty, and through the teens, human skin changes dramatically. The effects of heredity, sun, sleep patterns, and hygiene habits start to be seen by the age of twenty.

At maturity, men's and women's skin is remarkably different. Even in an individual, the skin can vary in texture and suppleness. One part of the face or body can be youthful and soft, another part dry and rough. As time passes the differences become more and more dramatic. By age forty, some women are still smooth and firm, whereas others look rough, loose, and sagging.

Your skin can make you look much older, or younger, than your chronological age. As you fight aging you might select weapons —treatments—appropriate to the present condition of your skin. To do this you'll have to find your skin's true age.

Each of the 24 questions below represents an hour in your "skin-clock." Check the statements that best describe the condition of your skin.

1. Oily surface and some blemishes, large pores with a tendency for blackheads.

1

2. Thick, dense skin with strong elastic bounce-back.
3. Medium, even-toned skin with smooth color.
4. Few problems with makeup or reactions to skin-care products.
5. Soft, firm skin with a bouncy elastic surface.
6. Medium texture, some resilience when pinched.
7. Open or enlarged pores in some areas of the face.
8. A tendency to freckles when exposed to sun.
9. Occasional patchy flakes and roughness.
10. Small lines on the outer edges of the eyes, or short horizontal lines across the forehead.
11. Normal pores, but a dry surface that feels tight and chapped in cold weather.
12. Blotchy uneven color, broken blood vessels, or freckles on the chest or sides of the face.
13. Makeup seems to cake, crawl, or vanish soon after it is applied.
14. Coarse or leathery skin that is rough to the touch.
15. Small wrinkles around the eyes and in the mouth area.
16. Dry or papery skin, tendency to enlarged pores.
17. Large freckles on the face, neck, and the backs of hands.
18. Extremely sensitive and irritable skin.
19. Thin, delicate skin with slow bounce-back if pinched.
20. Deep wrinkles, pouches, and sags.
21. Wrinkles on the bridge of the nose, earlobes, and chin.
22. Teeth appear longer and the lips thinner; the gums have receded.
23. Skin folds on the neck and the nape of the neck.
24. Wrinkles and creases cross each other, forming a network of lines; hair has thinned.

Your Skin Score

Each of the 24 hours on the skin-clock represents about two years of your skin life from the years eighteen through sixty-five—most of your adult life.

To score the quiz, add up the number of checks you made. Multiply the total number by 2. Add that number to the base young-skin number of 17 years of age. The number you get is your skin's true age, and ideally should be close to (if not the same as) or younger than your chronological age. If your skin age is too advanced for your liking, don't despair; you can make it younger.

Skin changes so quickly, it is easy to see how often you must reevaluate the skin-care and cosmetic products you use. A makeup that creates an allergic reaction, or a sleepless night, can add years to your appearance. And although your skin might seem to be stable and ageless in one part of your face or body, the aging process may have already begun in another place, necessitating immediate attention.

If You Want Your Skin to Lie about Your Age

When people describe beautiful skin they often liken it to baby's skin. But beautiful skin after childhood is possible, too. What is beautiful skin? It is smooth and velvety when it is touched. The surface is not puffy and soft, but it is firm and resilient. The texture is neither moist nor oily nor dry. It shouldn't be shiny enough to reflect light, but translucent enough to look bright and clear.

The pores of beautiful skin are small and almost, but not quite, invisible, and they are not dilated, even on the nose. A fine complexion has a slightly rosy or pinkish hue from active blood circulation.

Beautiful skin looks healthy, and any slight blemish quickly heals and disappears because the skin is well nourished and the basal layer of cells is always rapidly multiplying. It is the action of the cells and the underlying tissues and glands of the skin that keeps it looking young and strong, and keeps it beautiful. You cannot completely defeat aging, but if you understand it, you can keep the appearance of youth more years than you've dared to dream.

Think of your skin as a garment—one that will be your basic wardrobe throughout your entire life. As with all classics, although it might wear slightly, certain properties are never out of fashion, and you can preserve it and keep it looking new and fresh with a solid understanding of its nature and good care.

Adult skin seems to pass through four stages in about 40 years' time. Logically, delaying the onset of each successive stage can delay the aging of the skin. And different areas of your skin will age at different times. You cannot actually beat the clock of your own genetic biology, but you can squeeze every possible year, or month, or even day, of youth from your own genetic makeup.

The following background information about the four stages of skin will help you to identify more precisely what stage your own skin is in. You may find that you have an adolescent nose . . . and a middle-aged chin. You could then adjust your skin-care routine to deter further aging on your chin, while allowing your nose to slow down oil production and age slightly.

Young Skin (Teens–20's)

It can start as early as eleven, and keep going through your late twenties; your skin can be adolescent for two decades. The rapidly maturing skin is at its zenith in many ways during this time. It is strong, resilient, and it has amazing resistance. The skin is firm and taut with no sagging, wrinkles, or lines. It is at its elastic best. Usually the color is even, and although there might be a sprinkling of freckles, there are no broken blood vessels.

Adolescent skin is more moist than that of a child, and the oil glands are probably at their peak production level. When adolescent skin is blemish-free, it is as beautiful as it will ever be. But with puberty there is a chance that the body's rapidly changing hormone balance combined with active oil glands will result in clogged pores. The pores may become enlarged from the backed-up oil, and blackheads and whiteheads start to appear on the forehead, cheeks, and around the mouth.

Boundless energy keeps teenagers active in all kinds of weather. The sun seems a particular pleasure—it's a way of seeing and being seen. Exposure to the sun temporarily dries the surface of the skin and the peeling of the skin after a sunburn acts as a "skin abrasion," opening the pores and freeing them of clogged sebum. The skin during this time may seem indestructible—but the damage caused by the sun will show up in later years.

There is little need for creams and ointments during these years. What is needed is a method of keeping the skin clean and clear, without stimulating it too much, and without irritating it or spreading any skin infections that develop from the clogged oil pores. Wiping the skin with mineral oil (a no-no for older skin) can loosen the thicker natural oil that clogs the skin. But the mineral oil (or baby oil) should be followed by complete and careful mild abrasion, and then a complete washing with a mild soap.

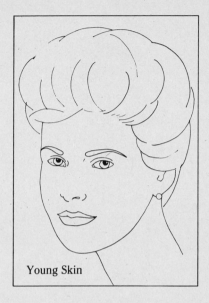

Young Skin

Avoid alcoholic fresheners after the soap. The skin can tolerate them better at this time than at any other time in life, but there is no reason to subject your skin to its strong effects. Use a medicated product for blemishes, but don't overdo. Several very gentle washings are better than strong medications that might encourage drying or allergic reactions.

Finish off every face washing with a spray of lemon-water (lemon juice mixed with water in a ten-to-one solution). It will keep the skin very acid and cut down on bacteria-inspired blemishes.

Check the responses that match your own skin:

— My skin is moist and oily.
— My skin seems to get dirty easily, almost as if it attracts dirt.
— My color is even, without darker areas, or light patches.
— My skin tends to blemish, especially during times of stress, or before menstruation.
— My skin is thick, taut, and resilient.

These are the hallmarks of adolescent skin.

Peak Skin (20's–30's)

Your body, your health, and your vitality are at their best at this time of your life. Your skin is also at its most perfect. It is smooth and very taut, and glowing with youth and beauty.

But, underneath, alas, the skin is starting the subtle changes that herald the aging process. One noticeable change during this time will be drier, less luxuriant hair.

Individual characteristics and inherited tendencies also start to show up at this time; if your mother has dry skin, this is the time that your skin might suddenly start to dry out. Or, even if you were just moderately oily in your teens, and you are from an oily skinned family, your skin might continue to be oily, and your pores are becoming more noticeable.

Because there is usually some slowdown in the oil production and the hormones of most people's bodies, the skin seems to stabilize during these years, and the skin is less prone to blackheads and bumps. The circulation of blood through the skin is strong and the heart and vascular system are healthy and young; there are no broken veins and few discolorations.

As you approach the end of this stage you may notice that small lines are starting to appear on the outer edges of the eyes. Although no other part of the skin is affected, the eye area shows age first because the skin is so thin. These tiny creases are almost indiscernible, but they are an indication of what is to come. The skin is thinning out all over and although it is still strong, taut, and resilient, there are slight changes in areas where the strain on the skin is the greatest. Smokers will notice these changes several years before nonsmokers; the eyes first, and then the sides of the mouth. Those who grimace or who have a heavy brow bone might also notice a line running across their forehead.

The color of the complexion may begin to look uneven. In very fair women there is a slight shift to a ruddy or pinkish hue. The soft, wholesome look of youth is blending into a rather outdoorsy look, and young adults tend to sunburn more easily than do teenagers.

About 20 percent of all the women in this age group will notice a bluish-brown darkening of some areas of the face. This is known as chloasma or melasma. It indicates excessive pigmentation in certain areas. Most of the discoloration is located in a masklike banner across the upper part of the face, but the blotches or darkened areas can appear on the sides of the face or the cheeks. This condition can be linked

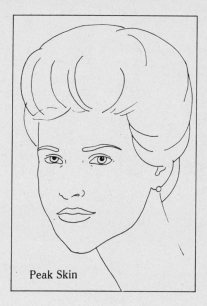

Peak Skin

with pregnancy or birth control pills, whether the pill is estrogen or pro-
gesterone dominant. The longer you're on the pill, and the higher the
dose of hormone in the pill, the more likely you are to develop this skin
discoloration. Dermabrasion, skin bleaches, and sunscreens can help
to get rid of these marks. You should wear sun-block makeup to protect
your skin at all times, as well as avoiding direct sunlight.

One of the most common skin-care problems in these young adult
years is perspiration. It is the body's way of regulating its temperature
and the most active, energetic sort of people are often bothered with the
problem. The body has more perspiration glands on the soles of the feet
and the palms of the hands than in any other place, but it is the under-
arm area that seems to encourage the most bacteria action, and so the
most odor. About a billion dollars a year are spent on deodorants and
antiperspirants (one stops the bacteria action and the odor, the other
stops the perspiration), and a large percentage of these products are
bought by young adults who are especially prone to stress-triggered perspiration.

Pregnancy is a common health-happening (rather than an illness) for
women during these years. Because of the hormonal changes in pregnancy there may be some temporary darkening of the face, the areolae,

and other areas of the body. Scars may darken and moles may enlarge. The stretch marks (striae) that can develop from any unusual change in weight often develop at that time. If your heredity is right, this can be kept under control with moisturizers that have cocoa butter in them, and also with applications of coconut oil.

The body skin may also show signs of change during the later years of young adulthood; cellulite suddenly may appear on firm thighs. The fat that is in large deposits in the upper leg and other areas makes this dimpling noticeable because the connective tissue under and around the fat starts to break down.

No matter what your chronological age, some parts of your skin may be at the young adult stage if these conditions describe your skin:

— My skin is usually clear and blemish-free.
— I have bumps or breakouts during stress periods.
— My skin seems dry, and sometimes I look tired and even haggard.
— I've noticed the first wrinkle that doesn't go away; no one else sees it, but it bothers me.
— Acne treatment products are too harsh and drying; they irritate my skin.
— The pores on my nose are oilier than on the other sections of my skin.

Plateau Years (30's–40's)

Age can leave its permanent mark on your skin as early as the second decade of life, or it can be retarded or delayed for almost 20 years—it all depends on you, your genes, your life, and your grooming. Unfortunately, when you become aware of the signs of aging, it may be too late; most of them may already be indelible. This is when you start to see the results of a "misspent" youth.

The skin at this time is rougher, dryer, and thicker on the surface but thinner overall than it was during the young-adult phase. Marks, warts, discolorations, broken veins, and allergic reactions can make the skin look ruddy or blotchy.

There is a dramatic decline in the oil production, and some glands cease to function entirely. The natural moisture has vanished and the skin is always dry, and often flaky. The skin suffers from the heat and cold without its fat pad to cushion it, and this also contributes to a ruddy and tough complexion.

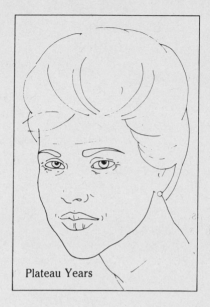

Plateau Years

There are definite wrinkles around the eyes now, and there is also a softening of the cheeks and chin. Lines that run between the nose and the mouth appear, and there is a slightly droopy look to the entire face. Disappointments, poor health, or even sleepless nights can show immediately on your face. Your skin doesn't seem to have the resilience that it once had. The pores may appear enlarged over the entire face, and the glossy feminine look of your young skin has almost disappeared.

As your hormone balance changes, and there is less estrogen in your body, there may be a tendency to gain weight, and you may even notice a personality change. Middle-aged women often find increased energy and drive, and it can be a time when you start new activities, or even a new vocation. You may have thought that this time—when your children and family are more able to take care of themselves—would be a time of more leisure for you, but you are restless and anxious to start something new. This higher energy level is fortunate, for this is also the time when you must change your grooming habits.

The hours in the sun, the weekends at the beach, the parties, and perhaps some health problems now are all too apparent. Many women find this time frightening; there are more changes in your body now than at any time since adolescence, and often less sympathy and support than you would like.

The acid and alkaline properties of the skin change, too. With the decreased activity of the oil glands, the skin becomes more alkaline. This dryness can cause itching and further irritation.

Moisture in the skin is also lost. The cells become weaker, and there is more evaporation from the surface. Moisturizers that "seal in" moisture help somewhat, but these give the skin a greasy surface. This moisture loss is most evident in the winter, when hours are spent indoors with artificially heated air, which is usually as low as 15 percent moisture. Look for a moisturizer that contains a moisture-attracting ingredient.

It's important now to faithfully continue a program of exfoliation. Abrading the upper thick layers of the skin will help moisturizers be more effective, and will minimize the sallow look caused by dead, tired skin cells.

Although exfoliation continues to be important, delicate treatment of the skin is essential. The connective tissue under the skin is weakening, and the collagen is weaker and becoming less resilient. Avoid brisk massages. Although strong facial treatments might make you look temporarily better, moving the skin away from the connective tissue can further the deterioration of the fat pads.

A note about makeup: The change in color and the change in surface texture of the skin dictate drastic changes in the makeup products you've been using. You should be using less, rather than more, on your face. Foundations have a tendency to sink into the wrinkles and cake around the eyes. It is very important to cleanse completely and to rid the face of any old makeup and to avoid any skin irritations. You need tender loving care; start giving *yourself* more of it!

Do you have partially or completely "middle-aged" skin?

— My skin flakes often, and there are rough areas.
— Small wrinkles have formed around my eyes, and especially around the bottom and outer edges of the lips.
— My upper eyelids are pouchy and less firm.
— I have noticed broken veins near my nose, or on my cheeks.
— My skin seems coarse and rough to the touch—no matter how much oil or cream I apply.
— There are some dark areas, and I seem to have more freckles on my skin.

— I look tired all the time—there is a softening in my chin and jaw and throat.

There is still time, even if your skin falls into this middle-aged category, to wake up those aging skin cells. With care, you can coax many more years of youth from your skin.

"Seasoned" Skin (50's– . . .)

It is only recently, with the long-overdue appearance of over-fifty high-fashion models, that this time of life has been reevaluated in terms of its own beauty. It is the time when the investments of your youth—be they in blue-chip securities or sound nutritional and living patterns—will now pay dividends. If you've made a lifelong commitment to skin care, this can be an attractive, if not glamorous, era of life.

In later years skin becomes increasingly delicate and is usually very dry, sensitive, and easily irritated. The texture can be papery instead of velvety; and dark-pigmented spots seem to appear daily on the face, forehead, hands, and chest. These marks can be very noticeable and will stand out even against a rough or deeply pigmented background.

Although the oil glands are small and not active in later years, blackheads and whiteheads may appear on the skin. It is because the pores shrink, and as they collapse the cells clog the tiny pores. The thicker surface skin also makes the journey of any oil and packed dead skin cells from the follicles difficult and slow, causing the blackheads.

The hair on the scalp and on the body thins and the growth of hair slows; but hair where you don't want it—on the face—may increase. Some of these changes in hair production are due to a decrease in ovarian function and a drop in estrogen level.

The drop of female hormones changes the texture of the skin, making it look more masculine; although the skin is now very thin and delicate, it no longer has the smooth, glossy appearance of typically "feminine" skin.

The most dramatic skin change during these years is the thickening of the outer layer, the epidermis, and the thinning of the inner layers, the dermis and the subcutaneous tissue. The connective tissues of the skin, collagen and elastin, become very weak and thin. They no longer hold and support the skin. As the collapse of the skin becomes more and more widespread, wrinkles and sags on the eyelids, the throat, and the cheeks become more evident. The lips thin noticeably, and the

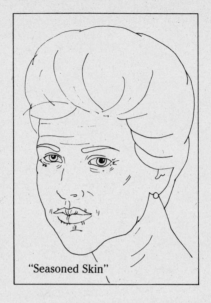

"Seasoned Skin"

gums also deteriorate so teeth are lost. Because the skin is so thin the veins look bluish and it makes the skin look gray and tired.

Older skin has a special need for moisture. Because there are few insulating fat pads, older people feel cold easily, and enjoy high room temperatures, which dry out the air, and make the skin even drier.

All of the changes that take place as the skin ages are natural, and although they are inevitable, they can be retarded for years if only a few simple precautions are taken. Preventive measures are most beneficial during the early years, but even later on, skin can be revitalized and rejuvenated. For example, the tendency toward ridged and brittle nails can be overcome with changes in diet at any age, and many of the discoloration marks on the skin and "liver spots" on the hands and face, and even tiny "cherry" angiomas (bright red bumps that often appear on the skin of people over fifty) can be removed by a dermatologist.

No matter what your age, any signs of skin deterioration should be treated as soon as you notice them. If any of the following characteristics apply to you, your skin is starting to show signs of age. There is still time to do something about it.

— My skin is dry and flaky.
— Small wrinkles have begun to form over the surface of the skin.

— My eyebrows seem to be coming closer and closer to my eyelids.
— My lips, even if I pucker for a kiss, don't look full.
— Small spots have begun to appear on my chest, neck, and hands.
— I bruise very easily, and often find a bruised mark on my arms or legs, but don't remember how it got there.
— There seems to be a thickening of the skin on the palms of the hands and soles of the feet.

No matter what your age you can look better (healthier). The knowledge that your skin is thinner and more vulnerable to bruises should make you careful about accidents. Good news: older skin, because it's more opaque, is less affected by sun damage.

How Old Is Your Skin?

Medical experts have developed chronological lists of the stages of aging that are reflected in the skin. These stages are so reliable that it makes it possible to predict when and where each aging sign may appear. The realities, depressing and relentless, are mapped out below. As you read through the descriptions, mark the box that best describes the qualities of your skin. After you've completed your chart, you will be able to tell which areas of your face are prone to premature aging.

Years

	18–27	28–36	37–45	46–54	55–63
Density	Thick, dense skin that bounces back immediately if pinched.	Strong, taut, resilient. Fat pads still adequate.	The outer layer of the skin thickens as the fat pad thins.	Skin's elastic fibers deteriorate and disappear. Dermis is thin and loses elasticity.	The outer layer of the skin becomes dry, thick, and opaque.
Color	Aging skin can start at this time. Use a sunscreen.	A slight shift in color toward a ruddy hue. No longer as even in tone or shade.	Ruddy with some tendency to blotchy sections.	Red cherry dots appear on trunk. Warts and warty moles appear.	Color is uneven and brown spots appear on the forehead and backs of hands.
Pigmentation	Even color with little difference in shading between face and body.	Darkening on forehead; mask during pregnancy.	Some freckles; mostly on cheeks, chest, and shoulders.	Heavy freckling, especially on forehead. Some freckles on hands.	Large brown spots on hand; loss of pigmentation in patches.
Muscle	Elastic, strong.	Strong and vibrant and more visible, giving the face definite character.	Varicose veins and other vascular problems start to appear.	Lines appear between eyes. Muscle mass has shrunk.	Cheeks sink in, making nose appear larger.
Texture	Smooth, tight skin. Velvety texture after washing. Slightly oily later.	Some sensitivity to perfume or other products, allergies are more evident.	Skin is coarse in appearance; pores appear larger. More sensitive to heat and cold.	Skin thins and is looser; when pinched it does not return immediately.	Papery texture of skin is evident; the skin seems lifeless.

	18–27	28–36	37–45	46–54	55–63
Blemishes	Black-heads and blocked pore problems.	Some large pores are evident in oily skin. Few black-heads form.	Wrinkles appear, pigment spots increase, skin looks blotchy.	Facial hair becomes more apparent. Broken blood vessels are evident.	Facial hair growth may increase, hair appears in nostrils.
Eyes	Dark circles appear. (Wear sunglasses to avoid early wrinkles.)	Laugh lines appear around the outer eye and lower lids.	Softening of the skin of the upper lid. Wrinkles of moderate depth around eyes.	Eyes puff and upper lid wrinkles; brows appear to lower and eyes become sunken.	Bags appear under eyes and wrinkles appear on sides of nose.
Mouth	Skin is thick and the gums are firm, forming a support for the mouth and cheeks.	First wrinkles appear around the outer corners of the mouth. Nasolabial fold from nose to mouth appears.	Facial expression around the mouth becomes set. Lips are plainly thinner.	The lips are paler and thinner. Wrinkles appear around the mouth.	Corners of mouth turn downward and cheeks sag and pouch.
Neck	Chin is firm and jaw is firm and taut.	Horizontal lines appear on the throat and base of neck, and jaw sags slightly.	Wrinkles in front of the ears at the neck are evident. Chin sags in profile.	Wrinkles appear in front of the ears and at the back of the neck. Skin on neck softens.	The base of the neck softens, and folds appear at the nape of the neck.

In the seventh and eighth decades of life, wrinkles crease over each other to form a network, and the scalp hair becomes sparse. The skin also becomes paper thin and seems lifeless. But there are some ways of keeping a youthful appearance for a longer period. Any cosmetic or cream that hydrates (adds water) to the skin's outer layers makes wrinkles less evident. Although cosmetic preparations cannot essentially change the nature of the skin, they can slow down the evaporation of water from within the skin and at the same time add a defensive coating to shield against any external irritants.

Many experts believe that aging is an expression of the inefficient metabolism of tissue. There could be many reasons for this: Endocrine gland malfunction or bad cellular nutrition are just two possible causes. In these cases, there is a possibility of reversing the aging process somewhat through glandular therapy and through additional nutrition to the cells.

The texture, color, and tone of the outer skin are only outward signs of the activity under the skin. Some dermatologists believe that in order to change or stop the aging process, therapy must be internal, penetrating the outer skin. There are ways to change and improve the skin's surface, however. Chemical peels and dermabrasion are possibilities. But an easier way is to gently exfoliate your skin daily, and in that way slowly, gently peel away the years.

2

Do You Know Your Own Skin?

Skin Facts

Your skin is not just a covering for your body; it is the largest and most visible organ you have. Your skin protects the body's bones and other organs by keeping them clean, by keeping them at a constant temperature, and by preventing them from moving around too much. Because skin is very resilient, it acts as a shock absorber for the delicate internal body. The skin also protects against attacks that we cannot see, such as ultraviolet radiation, microscopic particles and fungus spores in the air, and bacteria. The top layer of the skin is made of a thick protein that isn't soluble in water, so the rain, wind, snow, and other elements cannot penetrate it. The skin also prevents the soft and liquid inner person—the body is over 70 percent liquid—from leaking out.

The origin of human life was the sea, and it was in the sea that all animal skin started to develop. The ability to prevent the evaporation of water, and the oily coating of the surface of the skin with the low acid bacteria-fighting surface is probably linked to our aquatic origins.

In addition to its protective functions, the skin is also a very important sensory organ. It is the primary organ of one of our five senses, and helps to let us know how the outside world is treating us. It transmits all sorts of sensations, from heat to pain to pressure. There are more nerves in the skin surface than in any other organ except the human brain.

The skin is also a potent sexual organ. The outer layer, your skin, is what makes you look the way you look, and so determines to a large extent how attractive you are. And it is through the skin that we can be aware of the pleasure of a caress, a kiss, or the lightest, most delicate stroke.

The skin's oil glands are responsible for our own individual skin taste and odor. Some people just smell good to us, and others don't. Usually the smell is so subtle that we aren't consciously aware of it, but it emanates from the release of carbon dioxide from the skin's surface, and the release of hormones with the oil secretions of glands of the skin. Skin is very sexy.

If you live an active life, play tennis, have a job, or even walk rapidly, your body can produce as much as a quart of liquid a day in perspiration. That is released through the skin. That liquid is about 98 percent water, but it does contain some essential minerals and salts.

Your skin can account for about 14 percent of your total body weight. If you weigh about 130 pounds, that means that your skin might weigh over 15 pounds.

The skin of an average sized woman covers an area of about 20 square feet.

Like any organ, the skin is nourished by the blood. Poor circulation can lead to a dull, lifeless complexion. A good way of stimulating blood circulation is to fall in love, and to make love. If that is inconvenient, the next-best thing is to laugh heartily. Laughing not only improves circulation, but it also is minimally stressful to your skin and its support structure: when you smile and laugh you use only 13 muscles—when you frown you use almost all of your 60 facial muscles.

Despite its strength, the skin is vulnerable in many ways. Acne can strike at any age: It can be triggered by some medications, or from foods rich in iodine. Cosmetic products can also do the skin harm. Deodorants and some deodorant soaps, as well as some perfumes, can also encourage sunburns and brown spots on the skin. Beware of perfumed hand creams in the summer; they can cause smooth but splotchy fingers and hands.

Skin Structure

Human skin is made up of many parts:

- flat dead cells that form an outer shield
- sweat glands and tiny perspiration pores
- sensors for heat
- sensors for cold

— nerve endings to alert the body to pain
— pressure-sensitive nerve endings
— hair follicles
— small muscles woven through the skin layers
— rounded, water-filled skin cells

The skin is divided into two basic levels. The outer layer, called the *epidermis,* protects us from the outside world, and from evaporation and loss of body fluids. The inner layer, the *dermis,* contains the sweat glands and the oil glands and carries the blood supply and connective tissue that keep skin firm.

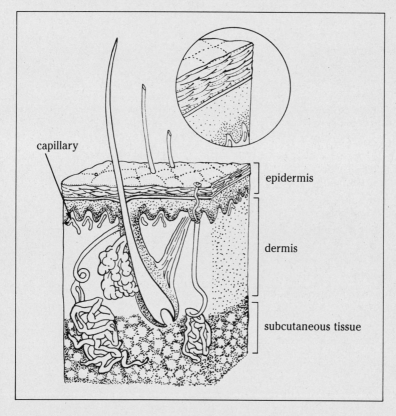

The epidermis, the upper layer, is about one-sixteenth of an inch thick over most of the body, except on the face, where it is even thinner. The skin is especially thin over the eyelids, the portion of the face between the nose and the mouth, and the throat. The skin on the backs of your hands is very thin, too. It is these areas that are covered with the thinnest epidermal skin that show age first. The thickest epidermal skin is usually on the palms of the hands and on the soles of the feet, especially the feet.

The dermis, the second level of the skin, is thicker than the epidermis. It accounts for the soft texture, the elastic quality, and the general shape of the upper surface of the skin. The dermis is usually about an eighth of an inch thick, but in some places—like the scalp, the palms, and the upper back and shoulders—it may be thicker.

There is a third level of tissue, a layer of subcutaneous fat that is under the skin. This layer is between the dermis and the internal body. The lower layers of the dermis and this under-padding of subcutaneous fat are not well defined and they vary in thickness.

All of these skin layers are loosely connected with strong bonds of collagen fibers. Through the bottom two layers are veins and capillaries that reach to every part of the skin. They carry blood to regulate the body temperature. There are small openings through the upper levels; these pores allow perspiration to flow onto the skin's surface. Other openings let hair, waste cells and oil move to the skin's surface.

When there is a breakdown in this fat layer, it seems to form lumps, making the outer skin look like "orange peel," a condition called cellulite. This third layer is composed of closely packed fat cells resting atop the muscles, and is what makes the feminine figure look smooth and graceful; its fat cells make the skin plastic and soft to the touch. The fat also acts as an insulator, absorbing shocks and preventing the loss of too much heat from the body.

It is the depletion of the subcutaneous tissue and fat, and the shrinking of the dermis, that make the skin thin and old. The thickening of the epidermal layer makes it look discolored and used. To keep skin looking youthful the uppermost layer, the epidermis, must be kept thin, smooth, and oily; and the underlayers, the dermis and the subcutaneous tissue, thick, soft, elastic, and firm. This gets harder and harder to do with the passage of time . . . but it can be done.

What the Skin Is Made Of

Water and protein are the major components of skin; together they make up almost 98 percent of the skin. The water in the skin cells contains some minerals and salts, but these constitute only about 1 percent of the total skin weight—sulfur, chlorine, iron, copper, calcium, and sodium are all present in minute quantities. Of these salts and minerals, it is sodium chloride we notice the most, because approximately one-third of the sodium chloride of the body is on the outer layer of the skin, left there as a waste product of perspiration. This salt absorbs water and acts as an antiseptic.

There are three kinds of proteins in the skin, and these proteins account for almost 30 percent of the skin's total composition. The proteins are keratin, found in the surface of the skin, and collagen and elastin, found in the dermis and connective tissues. Proteins are the essential part of every animal cell, including the skin's cells. They contain a high percentage of carbon and oxygen, and some nitrogen. The upper layer of the epidermis is mostly protein, but within that protein there is also some glucose, a natural sweetener.

Fatty acids, such as oleic acid (which is a colorless oil that turns yellow and brown when exposed to the air) and cholesterol, as well as other fatty substances, are a third important component of the skin. These oils keep the skin soft and pliable.

Small amounts of enzymes, hormones, and vitamins are also found in the skin. The most prevalent vitamins are A, B_6, B_{12}, and C. Check your diet to be sure to get some of each vitamin every day.

How Skin Reproduces

The epidermis, the outermost layer of the skin, is what the world sees. It is constantly changing. It is worn away by the elements, floated or sloughed away with washing, brushed away in contact with towels or clothing or complexion brushes, it is abraded away when it is scraped, and it flakes off and just flies away when it is no longer needed. If the skin didn't constantly renew itself we'd be skinless in about three weeks. But, in just about three weeks, the germinative layer of the epidermis of the skin produces new skin cells which make their way to the surface of the skin to replace the worn-out cells.

It is this outer layer that shows the discolorations, the blemishes, and most of the wrinkles to which skin is prone. It is responsible for scars and freckles. The epidermis is made of four layers of cells, and it is the bottom layer that produces new skin cells. This formation and moving upward of the cells is a continual process.

The cells reproduce by dividing, so some cells always remain on the bottom layer, where they act as a generative cell bank. When the cells are first formed, they are round, smooth, and filled with fluid, but as they move upward to the surface they change dramatically and become flatter and harder. The protein in each cell becomes more concentrated, and by the time the cells are on the surface they form a strong, almost waterproof shield. The technical word for this skin-growing and cell-maturing process is *keratinization*.

The cells of the uppermost surface of the epidermis are flattened and, like shingles on a house, they overlap each other. These cells are usually between 15 and 20 layers deep. Nature has made this layer very good protection; it is sometimes called the "horny" layer of the skin because the keratin is related to the substance that comprises your nails, your hair, and also the horns of many animals.

It is these thin, flat, hardened cells that you see when your skin peels after a mild sunburn. The horny layer contains no blood vessels and no nerve endings; it is nourished only by osmosis from tiny capillaries in the dermis. The only openings in the horny layer are the hair follicles, which also serve as openings for the sebaceous glands, and tiny perspiration pores. The oil flowing from those glands, and the skin cells they carry to the surface, prevent foreign objects from entering and invading the body through the skin.

On page 19 is a picture of the skin, showing the two basic layers of skin, the epidermis and the dermis, and also the fatty tissue underneath.

The Four Enemies of Young Skin

Your skin's age depends not only on when you were born, but also on your health and your genetic potential. Wrinkles, sags, and other signs of aging *can* be delayed somewhat if you follow some basic precautions, just as the aging process can be accelerated through careless or self-destructive behavior.

The aging of the skin is basically due to four factors:

The skin cells become toxic. The cells ceases to allow oxygen to pass through so there is a slowdown in the exchange of waste gases and life-giving oxygen. Without oxygen, the cells cannot live.

Poor blood circulation prevents the proper delivery of oxygen. Any organ that doesn't receive enough blood supply will not function correctly, and will eventually wither. All of the skin except the very outer portion, the epidermis, is fed by the blood supply. The blood continually brings oxygen to and carries away waste from the cells. The collagen and elastic tissue that holds the skin to the underlying tissues also must be serviced by the blood supply. A breakdown in the vascular system is signaled by broken capillaries, or thin spider lines. It means that the blood supply isn't even and continuous, and there is a blockage in the tiny hairlike capillaries that weave through the skin.

The cells become dehydrated and dry. The skin is composed of about 70 percent water, and it must remain moist in order to function properly. Aging is always accompanied by cellular drought. When you bake in the sun, walk in the wind, or subject your skin to freezing temperatures, the cells dry rapidly, and this drying causes them to die.

Even in the best conditions, like on a misty day in England, for example, dehydration takes place, and as you age, your skin becomes more and more vulnerable to dry climates, illness, and irritations, and the cells dehydrate very easily. Without water the cells pack down and the skin becomes thick, coarse, and rough. This loss of moisture most affects the dermis and the hypodermis (the underlying tissues). The upper layers are naturally dry and dead, so they change very little, they just become more dense. You can temporarily suffer this effect when you have a sunburn: the upper level thickens, and the lower levels dry out and die.

Shrinking of the under-tissue of the skin. The deterioration of the firm fat and tissue under the skin leaves the outer skin with less support and without that needed support, the skin ages rapidly. The general loss of elasticity and reduction of the size and number of active muscles in the muscle mass also leads to a loss of tone. The expression lines deepen when there is no cushioning under the skin, and the dry skin hardens, deepening the folds into wrinkles.

Of course the real "ager" is something you don't have much control over. Look at your mother, father, and other relatives: How have they aged? If you've inherited a thin, dry skin, you may have been blessed by very few blemishes during your teen years, but in your early thirties you might notice that your skin is thinning and coarsening. But because the skin grows continually, you can do something about this aging.

Your Skin and Your Body Systems

The skin is part of our complex body structure. The tissues, organs, and systems of the body must work together perfectly to keep us healthy. Everything—from pinched toes to a faulty liver—can rapidly reflect in the functioning of your skin. Some of the systems of your body that directly affect your skin are the circulatory system, the excretory system, the respiratory system, the muscular system.

The Respiratory System and Your Skin

With its high content of oxygen, air is almost as important as water in keeping your skin looking its best. When air is taken into your nose, it is passed by the warm vascular structures and cleaned of soot or pollution by very thin tiny hairs that line your nasal cavity. The longer your nose, the more thoroughly you can clean and warm the outside air. (Many anthropologists believe that the need to warm air before it enters your lungs is why people who have adapted to living in very hot climates usually have smaller noses than those who live in cold climates.)

After being warmed and cleaned the air passes along the inside of the throat and proceeds into the windpipe and finally into the lungs. The lungs are large, spongy half-cones that are made of air sacs. The walls of the air sacs are covered with a network of capillaries through which the blood cells continually flow. The cells give off carbon dioxide and then take in the oxygen that has been breathed into the body.

Your circulatory system is vitally related to the health of your skin, hair, and nails. Every living cell in your body breathes in its own way, and every cell must exchange carbon dioxide for oxygen to stay alive. Deep breaths bring more oxygen to your lungs and into your bloodstream than do shallow breaths, and deep breathing is important for the production of new skin cells.

Shallow breathing is associated with stress. Every mood you have is reflected in the way your breath is taken in and processed by the lungs, so your moods and emotions have a dramatic effect on cell function; many people forget to breathe when they're nervous, or they hyperventilate, and breathe too quickly.

If you're not getting enough oxygen into your lungs, you might be air-starved, and it will show on your skin. If you gasp when you talk, if your lips have a bluish cast, and if your face is ashen and sallow, you might be able to change your entire look through a small series of breathing exercises. Here is a routine that can oxygenate and reinvigorate your skin if you do it two or three times a day.

1. Close your mouth and draw into your lungs through your nose. Breathe in as deeply as possible.
2. Hold the air in your lungs as long as you can, or until you have counted to five, very slowly, in your mind.
3. Force the air out of your lungs and breathe out through your mouth. Do this as slowly as possible, and try to get every little breath of air from your lungs when you exhale.
4. Repeat, breathing in, holding your breath, and then breathing out through your mouth five times.
5. Relax and breathe normally.

Many people find that this breathing exercise has a little bonus built in. It seems to "clear the cobwebs" and makes you feel fresher, more energetic, and more mentally alert than before. Do be sure, though, that this exercise is performed outdoors where the air is clean, or in a room that is free of cigarette smoke. Breathing deeply near a smoker is almost as bad as smoking yourself.

Deep breathing is just one way to improve the health of your skin, but any activity that promotes higher blood oxygen levels will work. Try buying a small bag of balloons, and leaving them near the telephone, or someplace where you will be reminded to blow up a balloon every day. Another excellent way to nourish your skin is through aerobic exercise. The variations I have outlined below are simple, fast, and, best of all, effective.

Exercises for Better Skin

Tummy-Tight

1. Stand straight, and expel all the air from your lungs by breathing out through your mouth.
2. Bend over at the waist and place your hands, palms down, on your thighs.
3. Breathe in deeply. As you breathe in, pull up your stomach toward your chest.

4. Hold your breath for the count of three, and then relax and breathe out through your mouth.
5. Repeat three times. Do several times a day.

Panting-Pup

1. Open your mouth and exhale.
2. Pant—like an overheated puppy—for about 30 seconds.
3. Relax. Repeat three times.

Sipping-Air

1. Purse your lips as if you were drinking through a straw.
2. Slowly suck in the air, forcing it through your mouth, down into your lungs. (Notice how cool the air feels as it passes over your lips and tongue.)
3. Hold your breath as long as possible, and then exhale.
4. Relax. Repeat three times.

Bellows Breathing

1. Stand straight and expel all the air from your lungs by breathing out through your mouth.
2. Breathe in through your nose, filling your lungs as much as possible.
3. Blow the air out through your mouth forcefully in short bellowslike breaths. As you blow out, tighten your stomach muscles as much as possible.
4. Relax. Repeat three times.

There is really nothing that can give you a greater high than filling your lungs with air. The trillions of cells in your body are energized and invigorated with just one breath. The yogis have known the secret of deep breathing for thousands of years, and many of their astounding feats are based on the ability to control the air supply in their lungs. It helps improve your memory, too. But breathing is not the only way to get oxygen. You might also try "aerobic bathing." About 2 percent of the air that enters your body does come through the surface of the skin.

The skin also releases toxins in the form of perspiration. To be sure that the skin over your entire body has an opportunity to breathe and to be surrounded by air, try relaxing naked for about 10 or 12 minutes a day. If you lie on your bed, use pure cotton sheets because the natural fiber absorbs body toxins more easily, and its porous weave allows the air to circulate freely.

The Excretory System and Your Skin

Although we seldom consider the skin an excretory organ, it plays a key role in ridding the body of wastes and toxic products. Metabolism, a chemical process of converting foods and water into energy used by the body, also produces waste materials as side products. If these wastes are retained, they have a tendency to poison the body. Other organs that perform an excretory function are the kidneys, which excrete urine and rid the body of uric acid and used white blood cells; the liver, which discharges bile; the large intestine, which evacuates decomposed and undigested food; and the lungs, which exhale carbon dioxide.

The skin also takes part in the excretory process by eliminating salts and fluids through perspiration, which also keeps our bodies at a constant temperature. That is why it is very dangerous to cover the skin with paint, plastic, or even a very thick coating of cream that prevents the elimination of perspiration—and it's uncomfortable, too. Sebaceous glands in the skin coat the surface with oil, but the oil helps to carry away dead skin cells, and does not inhibit perspiration.

Fiber does not actually aid in digestion, although it is credited in helping in the elimination of waste material from the intestines. It speeds the food's passage through the digestive tract, and also aids bowel function. Some studies also indicate that a diet high in fiber will help to prevent hemorrhoids as well as some digestive diseases. The best way of getting fiber is in your food. Eating too much fiber can inhibit the absorption of calcium and zinc—two minerals that are vital for skin health.

Water is another essential component of proper excretory function, and is equally vital for healthy skin. Many people are afraid that drinking eight to ten glasses of water a day—or more—might cause water retention and make them feel bloated and tired. But medical experts firmly believe that drinking six to eight glasses of water a day is a basic guideline, and urge you to drink even more if you are exercising daily, to replace the fluid that escapes through perspiration during activity. The water you don't need, any "extra" water, will simply be eliminated. What can make you feel bloated is water that is retained in the body because it is combined with sodium, a substance you should try to avoid in excess. If you drink bottled beverages, check the label of your bottled water, or your carbonated drinks, to see if there is sodium in the drink—usually there is. Some foods are also high in sodium and will encourage your body to retain water. Avoid spicy and salty foods, and alcoholic beverages; they can make you feel thirsty, and contribute to the bloated feeling.

The Endocrine System and Your Skin

The endocrine system is a group of glands that acts as body regulators. They affect growth, reproduction, and your general health—depending on their secretions. These glands are specialized and vary in size and function, and they are triggered by the nervous system. The pineal gland and the pituitary gland, located in the brain, are part of this system; so are the thyroid, the adrenals, and pancreas. The reproductive glands that manufacture sex hormones which are needed for fertility and reproduction are also part of this system.

Your height, water retention rate, metabolism, and many other functions are regulated by the endocrine system. Any change in your hair growth or a dramatic change in the texture of your skin should be checked by a doctor.

The Nervous System and Your Skin

Neurology, the scientific study of the nerves and their structure and function, is becoming increasingly important. Your nerves affect every other system in your body. Every inch of your skin is supplied with nerve fibers. The nervous system controls and coordinates the functions of all the other systems, enabling everything to work together. There are three main parts to your nervous system: the brain, the spinal cord, and the nerves themselves. The best example of how nerves can affect your skin is your automatic response to a chill—"goose bumps." Your skin is covered with sensory cells; in one square inch there are more than 19,000 of these cells. They all carry messages about touch, heat, cold, smell, taste, and pain to the nerve centers in the brain. Stimulating the skin's nerves can be done very easily:

— by massage: touching, stroking, pressing, and slapping
— by electrical current: many facial treatments are based on passing a mild current through the skin
— by chemicals: acid or alkaline substances can irritate the skin and make it sensitive to the touch　　　·
— by exfoliating: scraping away of the skin's dead outer layer
— by heat, light, and exercise: factors that cause the blood to come to the skin's surface

All of these methods work, but many of these techniques are cumbersome to use. The idea of stimulating the skin is not new; and the use of exercise and stimu-slaps (see page 00) work better than many of these techniques. Any stimulation of the skin causes the muscles and blood vessels to expand, and the blood flows to the skin, which improves the blood's nourishment of the skin.

The Circulatory System and Your Skin

The heart is the center of your circulatory system. A muscular pump slightly smaller than your clenched fists, the heart works by contracting and relaxing in a pulsing movement, forcing blood from one section of the heart to another, and throughout the body. The oxygen-rich blood from the arteries goes through the body to service all the body's organs and tissues, while the carbon-dioxide-filled blood from the veins is passed through the lungs for purification.

The heart usually pumps between 60 and 70 times every minute. The rate at which the blood travels can be increased through exercise—up to five times its normal rate, but will naturally return to a slow, steady pace during rest or sleep. It takes less than two minutes for your blood to make the round-trip journey through your body. The same blood travels around and around, bringing oxygen and nutrients to the cells, including your skin cells, and carrying away waste, thus nourishing and purifying all parts of the body.

The skin's natural ability to reproduce cannot take place without a steady and continuous supply of blood. This constant circulation of the blood through the body is one of the secrets of a youthful skin.

Skin growth requires nutrients, oxygen, and the removal of waste; for this a blood supply is vital. The more blood, the more nutrients, and the better the potential for skin growth, which explains the importance of exercise to the skin: Exercise makes the heart pump faster, and brings more oxygen-laden blood to the surface of the skin.

Dr. John W. C. Bird, Director of the Bureau of Biological Research at Rutgers University, says:

> If you're not exercising there is much less blood in the skin and the body's periphery (fingers, toes, etc. and skin) compared with its central cavity (liver, stomach, etc.). With exercise more blood reaches the periphery, the skin receives more nutrients, and the exchange of oxygen is increased, and there is a release of perspiration. All of this is tremendously beneficial to the skin.*

Gravity boards, yoga, and even "mind-control" have been used to increase or redirect blood flow. All of them work—but exercise does it better, and faster, with the added benefit of strong muscles and bones.

Exercise speeds up the pace at which blood circulates throughout the body, and it also acts to keep all the tiny blood vessels that permeate the dermis open and invigorated, making the skin rosy in color.

Have you noticed how warm you get when you exercise? Even in the dead of winter joggers seem immune to arctic blasts! Any physical exertion generates heat, and that heat, carried by the blood supply, is released through the skin, raising the skin's surface temperature. When you participate in active exercise, your overall body temperature rises, and your surface skin temperature can rise as much as 5°—from about 88°F to about 93°F. When the temperature on the surface of the skin rises, it also affects the bacteria that live on the surface of the skin, and because some of those bacteria cannot withstand the change in temperature, they perish. The skin of a well-exercised person is warm, engorged with blood, bathed in perspiration, and inhospitable for many disease-carrying bacteria.

Dr. Albert Kligman, professor of dermatology at the University of Pennsylvania School of Medicine, has said, "Temperature is very important in determining the condition that the skin is in." He cites Russian reports of athletes, which indicate that the collagen content of the skin goes up and the skin becomes more dense when the athletes are in intensive training. "With exercise and the increased nutrition of the skin," Dr. Kligman notes, "you may lay down more dermis. The rate at which collagen is produced is probably temperature dependent."

Other medical experts are also interested in the effects of exercise on

*From "Exercising for Healthy Skin," by Jane Ogle, *The New York Times Magazine*, December 6, 1981.

the growth of skin tissue. Dr. James White of the University of California at San Diego compared samples of skin from a matched group. He found that those who exercised had denser, stronger, and thicker skin than those in the sedentary control group. He has also found that people who exercise regularly have fewer wrinkles than those who do not exercise. (But, he has noted that exercising in the sun can be worse than not exercising at all!)

One last way that exercise can benefit your skin is by helping you fight stress. Stress can cause a tightening of the muscles, and that can constrict the flow of blood to the skin's surface. Through exercise, those tense muscles will relax, and the blood supply to the skin will increase—a surefire way to younger, healthier-looking skin.

Blood Food

You're as young as you look and you're as young as you feel, and you look and feel exactly the age of your arteries. If you can keep your vascular system and the network of arteries and veins in your body smooth and elastic, your skin will be well-fed and glowing, and you will have boundless energy. All the health food diets and all the exercise will do you very little good if your arteries are not resilient and open.

The arteries are constructed of flexible tissues. They are elastic pipelines made of three layers: The outer layer is a protective coat that also carries the nerves and blood vessels which supply the arteries themselves. The middle layer is thick, smooth, and muscular. The inner layer is a thin, smooth lining. As the arteries branch out through the body they become smaller and thinner so that they are finally threadlike, with very delicate walls. These thin walls allow body fluids to pass through; that is why your arteries are so important in the growth of new skin cells.

One of the traditional vascular decloggers is a mixture of milk, honey, and brewer's yeast. Whether or not it can actually unclog your arteries is unknown, but it is healthful, and delicious on breakfast cereal. Try this recipe:

1 tablespoon brewer's yeast (powdered type)	½ teaspoon honey
	Enough yogurt to make
½ cup skimmed milk	a cupful

Mix and use according to your own taste. (Note: Yeast can trigger acne.)

5-Minute Skin-Gym

The good news about the relationship between exercise and the condition of the skin is that the exercise doesn't have to be long, complicated, and strenuous. The best exercise is movement which unkinks the muscles and stimulates a steady, strong, and even flow of blood to the extremities—the fingers, feet, and the face and scalp. For office workers and millions of other people who don't have much opportunity to move around during the day, or to participate in muscle-relaxing sports or activities during the day, all you need is five minutes spent in doing these simple rhythmic motions.

1. *Stand up, stretch, and yawn:* Rise on your toes, arms over your head, reach upward and try to touch the ceiling, then outward and try to touch the walls. Drop arms, stand flat.
   Repeat 5 times.
2. *Stomach pull; buttocks lift:* Tighten stomach muscles and pull in as hard as you can. Relax. Tighten buttocks muscles and pull up as hard as you can. Relax.
   Repeat 5 times.
3. *Torso swing:* Bend at the waist, drop down, and let your arms dangle toward the floor. Sway back and forth so that your right hand passes your left foot and vice versa, twisting your torso as you swing. Stand straight.
   Repeat 5 times.
4. *Hip thrust:* Place hands on the hips. Rotate your lower torso first, thrusting forward, then to the right, then to the left, and finally arch your back, pushing your lower torso backward. (Be sure your shoulders are held still and level to get the best effect.) Relax.
   Repeat 5 times.
5. *Shoulder shrug:* Relax arms, and let them dangle at your sides. Lift one shoulder as high as possible, trying to touch your ear. Relax. Lift the other shoulder to touch the other ear. Roll the head around, letting it flop forward and backward. Relax.
   Repeat 5 times.

These movements are not really exercises in the traditional sense. You don't have to change clothes, or get warmed-up, or do anything unusual. Try to repeat one or all of these stretches several times during the day. You'll find that you're energized because you're loosening and flexing more than straining. You'll also find that you are becoming agile and more graceful, and your skin will appreciate the increased blood supply.

The Muscular System and Your Skin

The skin rests on tissues and muscles that cover our skeleton frame. Massage and stimulation to the muscles, as well as exercise that is designed to build the muscles, have been used as methods of benefitting the entire body—and of firming the skin. The muscles are the organs of movement, and we have more muscles in our face and neck than any other animal—the muscles, over fifty-five of them, allow us to communicate through expressions.

The skin of the face and neck is thinner than other skin on the body, and the muscles of the neck and face are very delicate because they are small and composed of thin, fine muscle fibers. These muscles are easily stretched, strained, and abused. The muscles of the face (remember, there are dozens of them) easily lose elasticity, become slack, and the tendons that attach them to the small facial bones become loose as the fat pads under the skin shrink with age. All of these factors lead to muscle sags, and that leads to skin sags, flabbiness, wrinkles, and soft pouches.

Moving the muscles of the face must be done very gently, and very slowly and carefully. But before attempting to move your muscles to prevent them from atrophy, and to stimulate as active a blood supply to the face as possible, you should know where the muscles are, and what sections of the face and skin some of the major muscles control.

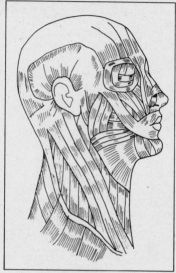

The Muscular System

Forehead: The frontal muscle, a wide, flat muscle, covers the entire forehead. When you contract the forehead muscles, the skin shifts, squeezes together, and forms a horizontal wrinkle across the forehead.

Eyelids: A round, doughnut-shaped muscle controls the movement of the eyelids and is involved in the way wrinkles form about the eyes. Wrinkles from the contraction of this muscle show up as crow's-feet.

Cheeks: A series of ribbonlike muscles that weave in and out of the cheeks and allow you to smile; they are called the zygomatic muscles. When you contract them, the corners of your lips move upward.

Mouth and lips: A round doughnut-shaped muscle controls the mouth and lips. When this muscle contracts, the lips compress inward, or they blow a kiss outward. The quadratus labia is the muscle on the upper part of the lip that can pull the upper lip toward the nose. There is also a muscle in the lower lip that allows you to pout.

Jaws: Muscles on the side of the face that allow you to chew. They raise the jaw and allow it to move forward and from side to side.

Neck: The muscles that cover the spinal column allow you to move your head, to bow, and to control the rotation of your head on your shoulders. Another set of muscles moves the shoulders and your arms. Flailing your arms around or lifting them over your head stimulates the blood supply to all the muscles of the face and head.

Small muscles on your nose allow you to dilate your nostrils, and many other small muscles that permit subtle nuances of movement and expression.

Muscle-Massage,
the "Professional-Facial" Way

You'll need a warm, private, well-lighted place where there is easy access to water—your bathroom is ideal. Gather together the following equipment and materials:

- a large bath towel
- a terry-lined shower cap
- a small sponge (I like natural sea sponges)
- facial tissues
- an oily face cream, or thick animal or vegetable oil
- a teaspoon of lemon juice
- a tray of ice cubes
- soothing music.

Take off all your clothes and wrap yourself in the large bath towel, but leave your arms and shoulders bare. Cover your hair with the shower cap.

Wash your hands and face carefully. Rinse your face well. Apply the oily cream or vegetable oil to your shoulders, neck, throat, and face. Apply from bottom to top, shoulders to forehead, always stroking upward.

Shoulders

Breathe deeply and loosen shoulders by shrugging several times. The shoulder muscles that run from the neck to the joint of the shoulder and arms need to be kneaded. Cross your arms in front of your chest, and place your right hand on your left shoulder. Knead and hack the muscles; work slowly to stimulate the circulation as much as possible. Your hands should work from the outer edge of the shoulder toward your neck.

Stretch the fingers of your hands and work down the middle of the back, then work upward, patting, kneading, and hacking gently up your neck to your hairline.

Relax arms by letting them drop.

Repeat 4 times.

Jaw and Chin

The muscles of your neck run along your jawbone and are attached to your cheekbone in front of the ears. Starting on the side of the chin, work toward the earlobe.

Use the knuckles of your fingers, move one hand above the other and "step" your hands from chin to ear along the jawline.

Pat the skin under the chin and along the lower jaw with the back of your hand.

Relax by letting them drop.

Repeat 4 times.

Mouth

With your fingertips, start below the corners of the mouth and gently tap the skin on the outer corners of the mouth, and then work upward over the expression lines that run from nose to mouth.

Using a light piano-fingering motion with the middle and fourth fingers, work upward toward the corners of your nose.

Relax arms by letting them drop.

Repeat 4 times.

Eyes

The skin around the eyes is loosely attached to the underlying muscles; that is the reason that the skin on the upper lids seems to droop so early in life. Use your most delicate and lightest touch in this area.

Tap *very gently,* circling the eye with feathery taps from the temple to the inner corner of the eyes, first over the upper eyelid, then just as gently under the eye. Move in feathery strokes.

Relax the arms by letting them drop.

Do not repeat.

Forehead

The muscles of the forehead run vertically from above the eyes and bridge of the nose to the scalp.

Start above the bridge of the nose, using tapping motions of the fingertips; work upward and outward. Hold your hand level with your forehead and tap as if on a very stiff piano or typewriter keyboard.

Relax arms by letting them drop.

Repeat 4 times.

Your skin should be pink-hued and glowing from the stimulation of your tapping fingers. Rinse the excess oil off your face with warm water, and then continue to rinse, gradually cooling the rinse water by changing the mixture of hot and cold.

Fill the wash basin with cold water and add the tray of ice cubes. Add the lemon juice. Dip the sponge into the icy water, squeeze out the excess, and pat the icy, wet sponge gently against the skin. Go over the shoulders, neck, and face until the skin tingles.

Young Neck—Young Voice

As you age your voice changes slightly. This seems to happen at very much the same time as those wrinkles and sags appear on your neck. As you age all your muscles and tissues become less resilient, and the muscles around the vocal cords are no different. The length of the vocal cord and the tension on the cords accounts for the vibrations and the pitch that make up your voice. If you want to keep your voice—and your neck—smooth, lilting, and attractive, you can do these simple exercises to keep the muscles taut and the vocal cords and neck smooth and young.

Head-Roll

Drop your head forward so that your chin is near the top of your chest. Roll your head around to the right, and then to the left. Try to get your ear to rest on your shoulder (a goal more than a reality). First the right shoulder, then the left. Then roll your head backward so that your chin points to the ceiling. Relax by lifting your head to its normal position. Repeat every few hours if you sit at a desk, looking down; or if you work at a typewriter, word-processor, or computer.

Chin-Ups

Cover your upper lip with your lower lip. Bring your lower lip as far as possible toward your nose. Relax. Cover your lower lip with your upper lip. Bring it down as far as possible, trying to cover your chin. Relax. Repeat several times whenever you can think of it.

Eye Gymnastics

Food, air, and exercise create a strong vital blood flow, bringing blood to where it is needed. One of the places it is needed most is the area around your eyes, and only eye exercises can increase the circulation to this area. Six strong muscles that are like thin strings are attached to your eyeball; these are the muscles that must be exercised to improve blood flow. The following simple eye drills will take only a few minutes a day:

1. Turn your head left, then right, then left and right; your gaze should follow the movements of your head. Keep turning so that your focus is at a point over your shoulder. Repeat 12 times.
2. Hold a coin (a dime is a good size) about 6 inches from the tip of your nose. Focus on it. Switch your focus to a point in the far distance. Repeat 12 times.

If you do close work, or if you use a computer terminal, remember to do these exercises at least twice a day or more. *Exercise rather than rubbing your eyes*—rubbing the delicate eye skin is very damaging.

When your eyes do get tired or irritated, this exercise, developed by a noted medical expert, will help to relax the muscles around your eyes.

Stand in front of an object or picture. Focus on the object as intently as you can. Stare for a moment. Then, close your eyes and cover your closed eyes with your cupped palms. (Do not put any pressure on your eyelids or eyeballs.) Gradually open your eyes inside the cupped palms. All you will see is black. Stare into the darkness and breathe deeply. Count slowly to 10. Close your eyes. Drop your arms. Relax.

You'll notice your eyes are refreshed and you can focus more easily. Changing your focus also helps. After close work, focus on some distant point. If you've been driving and scanning the horizon, focus closely. These changes in focusing will change the shape of your eyeball and put tension on different muscles. It will relax other muscles, and you'll notice your entire face looks less tense or haggard. Eyestrain causes squint lines at the outer edges of the eyes and the muscles of your neck and shoulders tighten when you strain or squint, decreasing the blood supply to your entire head and neck.

3

Your Face-Friends

Skin-Care Habits

Sun, wind, time, and a host of other agers are always at work, weakening your skin and making the surface rough and dry. But there are defensive and offensive weapons available. Use them all, or select the ones that seem best suited to your life-style. Most good skin-care habits will do more for your skin than costly skin-care products or cosmetics. Keeping your skin young is similar to dieting and exercise—you must acquire habits of skin care that are automatic.

Sleep and Your Skin's Health

If you've recently endured a sleepless night, or even a restless night, you know what effects those few hours of deprivation can have on your skin. At twenty you can recoup your energy easily, but by forty it may take several days to a week to get over that dragged-out feeling—and for your skin to look clear and healthy again. Sleep is vital because the nutrients that help new skin cells to form are not assimilated properly without sleep. Another reason is that much-needed oxygen is brought to the skin best during sleep.

Without food, and the oxygen needed to convert that food to skin tissue, the natural growth of the cells slows, or even ceases completely. Here are some sleep-seeking ideas that will help you get the sleep you need for skin health.

— Arrange your sleep place (bed, sofa, etc.) in a dark area away from light or reflected glare from mirrors or shiny surfaces.

— A box spring mattress is most comfortable for most people. Some people can sleep peacefully on the floor, or in a hammock, but these generally are not the most comfortable sleeping surfaces.

— Use a small, flattish pillow or a baby pillow with only a pure cotton or linen pillowcase. If your pillow is large or too soft, it will block your breathing. If the pillow is too high, your neck is bent, your face curls toward your chest, and you can't breathe easily. The natural fabric on the pillowcase absorbs perspiration more easily and remains cool and comfortable.

— Keep your feet and arms warm. During sleep your blood supply leaves your outer extremities and collects in your torso. Blankets and quilts that are soft and fluffy conserve body warmth without weight.

— Be sure that your food intake in the hours before bedtime includes calcium, magnesium, vitamin D, and vitamin B_6. "Calcium," wrote food expert Adelle Davis, "can be as life-saving as an oxygen tent."

Calcium for a Good Night's Sleep

Calcium is a mineral that helps promote a soothing alkaline-acid balance in the blood and allows you an undisturbed, restful sleep. A constant supply of calcium is needed in the circulating blood for building bone and for controlling the electronic impulses transmitted through nerves. If the calcium supply falls below normal levels, the nerves become tense, and as a result muscle cells contract. Without enough calcium your muscles contract as you sleep, causing spasms, or charley horse cramps.

The older you get, the more calcium you need, because your ability to absorb this essential mineral diminishes with the years. During menopause women frequently have difficulty sleeping, and over a period of time their bones become fragile as calcium is drained from their bones and tissues. It may be that the traditional cure for sleeplessness—a glass of warm milk—has some scientific foundation! Here is a folk remedy that is a calcium tonic:

COUNTING SHEEP

1 whole banana, sliced   1 tablespoon honey
½ cup yogurt   sprinkle of cereal

Mix everything together in a bowl. (The slices of the banana represent the little sheep.) Count each slice as you eat it, and chew very slowly and very carefully. The nitrogen, phosphorus, and calcium in the banana form a combination that satisfies; it is quickly assimilated into the bloodstream and promotes a feeling of calm and relaxation. The banana is also a source of vitamins A, B-complex, niacin, essential minerals, some amino acids, and vitamin C. The yogurt provides calcium and the honey contributes a feeling of well-being.

Understanding Sleep

Sleep was once a complete mystery; even now it is not completely understood. Much of what scientists know about sleep comes from connecting electrical monitors to the bodies of sleeping people. These devices record the tiniest electrical signals from the brain, the eye movements beneath the closed lids, and even the movement of the facial muscles.

The average woman lies in bed fewer than 15 minutes before falling asleep. Gradually, as she sinks into a twilight zone and becomes less aware of everything around her, muscles relax, and her blood pressure, heart rate, and body temperature then begin to decrease. This period is called Stage 1, the "alpha" period of sleep.

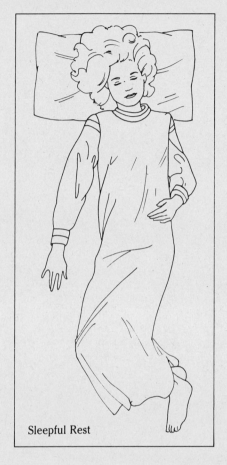

Sleepful Rest

After a few minutes, another sleep pattern emerges; it is called Stage 2, and it is the first level of true sleep. Within 15 minutes, the brain and body slow down still further, and the sleeper enters Stage 3 of sleep, and later Stage 4, which can be recorded in slow, even waves of the graph that displays the signals from the electrodes attached to the sleeper.

In Stage 4, the deepest sleep, the cells of the cortex (the top layer of the brain) are no longer firing along complex dispatches to the body in the way they do during waking hours, or even the slower signals of the first stages of sleep. Instead they send waves of rhythm. The senses are turned off, and memory is blocked. The heart rate, blood pressure, and breathing rate decrease, and a different kind of body activity takes place.

The new activity is the manufacture of hormones, enzymes, and other body chemicals that must replace what is used during wake-time. The skin needs these hormones, and it also needs the inactivity of this deep stage of sleep to grow properly. It is during the night, and during this deep stage of sleep, that the skin creates most of the new skin cells. If you're doubtful, just spend a few sleepless nights and then notice the deterioration of your skin.

The deep sleep, Stage 4, usually starts about 30 to 60 minutes after the onset of the first, or "alpha," stage of sleep. About 90 minutes after the onset of sleep the body usually rouses, the sleeper shifts position, and may come from the deep sleep back through the other stages. The entire night is spent in going back and forth from a light sleep or almost waking stage to deep sleep.

After about an hour and a half, the Rapid Eye Movement (REM) stage of sleep, which is between the waking and the second stage, takes place. The eyes dart around under the closed lids and the breathing becomes irregular. REM sleep is when the brain starts to dream.

In childhood there are long periods of the deep stage of sleep, and as a young adult, about 20 percent of sleep time is spent in the deep Stages 3 and 4. But with age, the time spent in deep sleep—the time that many important hormones and enzymes are manufactured—almost disappears. When the deep-sleep stage disappears, the chemicals are not manufactured. The altered sleep pattern is another contribution to the aging process. Interestingly, one of the most consistent things about all people is that their sleep patterns at certain ages. Babies fall into a deep sleep almost immediately, and older people enjoy this complete surrender less and less as they age.

The 8-Hour Facial and
Complete Beauty Treatment

It seems a shame that the time spent in sleep, while beauty-giving in it-self, is not completely devoted to very intensified skin-bolstering. But it can be, with just a bit of forethought. Suffuse your slumber with skin-building, protective, and healing unguents. Here's how:

— Gather together a man's cotton T-shirt, or a long T-shirt of your own, a white handkerchief or terry band to protect your hair, white cotton socks, and a pair of old white cotton gloves.

— Wash and set your hair, or arrange your hair the way you usu-ally would at bedtime, and wrap it in the cotton kerchief.

— Take a short (not more than 10 minutes) warm bath, and after sitting in the tub long enough to soften the skin, slough off the dead cells with a loofah or a soft brush, or a handful of abrasive grains such as oatmeal.

— Rinse your skin carefully and completely. Without drying off, spray yourself with a mixture of 1 teaspoon lemon juice and 1 pint of tap water.

— Coat your body with coconut oil and avocado oil, mixed in equal measure. Don't forget your legs, feet, arms, wrists, and hands. Then cover yourself with the old T-shirt.

— Add an extra coat of coconut oil and avocado oil on the feet and hands, and then on go the socks and gloves.

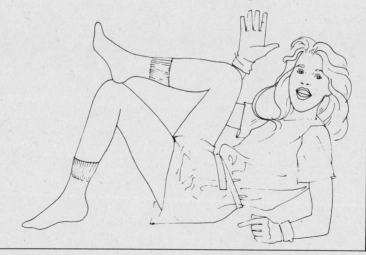

Although regular, undisturbed sleep gives your skin the time it needs to replenish itself, there is no reason why you can't make use of this sleep time with some easy-to-make nighttime beauty treatments for the face and other "trouble spots." Make several "treatment pocket-masks" by folding a woman's cotton handkerchief in half, and attaching an elastic or ribbon to either end. I like a lacy handkerchief because it looks pretty. You can use the little mask over your eyes, mouth, or under your chin, and you can use more than one mask if you want a more total treatment. When you are finished using the mask, you can wash it easily and it will be fresh and clean. If you iron the handkerchief with a hot iron, it will be sterilized before using it again.

To soothe puffy eyes: Fill the two pockets with tea bags that have been steeped in hot water, squeezed free of excess liquid, and then cooled. Chamomile tea is the best, but other teas, including India and China teas, work well, too. (Tea can stain, though, so don't use your best hankie with this treatment, and make sure you choose one that can be safely bleached.) Tie the tea compresses over your eyes, and drift off to sleep.

For thick lashes: Fill the two pockets with cotton that has been soaked in castor oil, and tie them over your eyes. In the morning your lashes will be longer and lustrous. Continued use of castor oil on the lashes will encourage new growth and make them longer and stronger.

For a soft, smooth throat: Coat your throat with olive oil, or some other vegetable oil, and tie the handkerchief around it. The mask will keep the oil on your neck, and will prevent the oil from getting on your sheets.

For smooth, soft lips: Coat your lips with petroleum jelly, and cover the mouth area with a rich vegetable oil. Place the mask over the mouth, and tie in the back of the head. Your lips and mouth will be soft and your upper lip and chin area will enjoy a treatment that lasts all night.

To smooth rough elbows and knees: Using an old sock, cut the toe section out so that the sock forms a tube. Rub a rich oil (avocado works well) on your knees and elbows. Using a pair of socks for the knees and one for the elbows, cover them carefully and allow the oil to stay on the skin during the night.

Use a small or flat pillow while you're getting your "beauty sleep," and be sure the window is open slightly and there is good ventilation in the room. When you're all decked out in parts of socks, handkerchiefs, gloves, and T-shirts, you'd probably best sleep alone. This is a private beauty routine that should be your secret.

Turn Your Skin Pink with a Yellow Fruit

In addition to a restful night's sleep, vitamins and minerals, the essential components of good nutrition, are vital to healthy skin. One of the most basic of these is vitamin C, a nutrient that encourages healthy connective tissues which bind all the individual cells together, and compose cartilage, veins, and ligaments. The red blood cells carry oxygen to each of the individual body cells, and vitamin C from something like lemon juice, a prime source of this vitamin, carries hydrogen and other ingredients needed for metabolism and nourishment of the skin's tissues. Lemons have always been popular as a "beauty aid," and with good reason.

The juice of the lemon can encourage new skin growth. Once the nutrients of the lemon juice are assimilated into your bloodstream the amazing skin-growth cycle begins. The nutrients help the skin's own ability to shed and replace the outer layer of skin with fresh new cells. The clinging of the old or dead destroyed cells to the skin inhibits healthy skin functioning, and slows down the re-forming process of the new cells. This is one of the prime causes of old-looking skin.

Used as a clarifier, lemon juice helps to tone the skin and invigorate it. The new cells make the skin always fresh and smooth. This stimulation seems to speed up skin metabolism, and it also leads to relaxing of the muscles. The action of the nutrients of the lemon encourages a melting away of any clogged grime or wastes that contribute to rough, dull-looking skin. The enzymes also normalize the acid/alkali balance on the skin, which makes all the difference between glow and gray. A word of warning: some people have noted an adverse reaction to lemon juice; it is too acid for their skin. Start by mixing lemon juice with water. Use a solution 1 part lemon juice to 10 parts water.

Here's a lemon Skin-Sip recipe that tastes great and will help you look terrific:

Mix 2 tablespoons lemon juice with 1 cup of tomato juice; sprinkle with basil, and top with a sprig of parsley. Cheers!

Vitamin B₃, a Natural Rouge

In treating the elderly and people who suffer from balance or inner-ear problems, many medical experts prescribe niacin, which opens narrowed blood vessels. The use of this B vitamin has an interesting side effect: It makes patients look better as well as feel better. The reason for the success of the vitamin treatment cannot be pinpointed, but vasodilatory action of nicotinic acid (niacin) is well known, and the vitamin has been used for many years just for this purpose. It is a happy coincidence that the flush and dilation of the blood vessels bring blood to the surface of the skin, causing a rosy glow and fresh complexion.

Nicotinic acid has at least one other effect, besides the dilation of the blood vessels. It is the reduction of blood cholesterol level, if taken in very high dosage. If you take between 50 to 100 milligrams of niacin about 20 minutes before each meal, you'll be getting the best effect from this potent vitamin. As with any large dosage of vitamin, it is wise to check with your doctor first.

Skin Solutions

Problem	Solution
Dry, flaky skin; rough, scaly texture	*Vitamin A:* Milk, cod-liver oil, eggs, carrots, tomatoes, sweet potatoes, liver, kale, cantaloupes
Rough, easily irritated skin, insects seem to be attracted to you, edema, sweating	*Vitamin B$_1$* (Thiamine): Found in peanuts, beans, pork, ham, internal organs (beef heart), grains, nuts, yeast
Rough texture, scaling, flakes, and poor circulation, cracks on lips	*Vitamin B$_2$* (Riboflavin): Found in oatmeal, yogurt, leafy greens, dairy products, kidney
Sallow skin, dizzy spells, poor circulation, bluish fingertips, circles and shadows under the eyes, pellagra	*Vitamin B$_3$* (Niacin): Found in liver, poultry, fish, brown rice, seeds, nuts, yeast
Scaling, psoriasis, excessive dandruff, nervous facial tics, sagging skin	*Vitamin B$_6$* (Pyridoxine): Found in bananas, wheat germ, whole grains, brown rice
Skin lesions, grayish hue, difficulty in sleeping, dull hair, skin, and eyes	*Biotin:* Found in wheat germ, peanuts, liver, egg yolks, dark green vegetables
Graying, drab-colored hair, skin allergies	*Para-aminobenzoic Acid:* Found in organ meats, liver, yeast, nuts, whole grains
Blotchy skin with dark patches, broken blood vessels, spider capillaries	*Vitamin C:* Found in oranges, lemons, strawberries, brussels sprouts, broccoli, green peppers, watercress (Look for bright-colored foods.)
Bones, teeth, and muscles are weak and thin	*Vitamin D:* (essential for bones and teeth); Found in fish and fish liver oils; sunlight, bananas

Problem	Solution
Skin and hair looks old, low sex drive	*Vitamin E* (the antisterility vitamin); Found in wheat germ, whole grains, all vegetable oils
Tough skin, poor texture, uneven tone, pale, graying color	*Vitamin F:* Found in vegetable oils and mayonnaise
Black-and-blue bruises, poor clotting, sallow skin tone	*Vitamin K:* Found in cabbage, cauliflower, spinach, leafy greens, corn, tomatoes, eggs, strawberries
Slow growth of nails, thin hair, low energy, bruises easily	*Protein:* Found in milk, meat, cheese, chicken, fish, lentils, peanuts, wheat cereals
Pale, thin skin, pale nails, bluish lips, circles under eyes	*Iron:* Found in lima beans, liver, oysters, lentils, almonds
Restless sleep, cramps, nervous tics, slow healing and blood coagulation	*Calcium:* Found in broccoli, cheese, yogurt, milk, eggshells (edible although not tasty), sardines (with the bones)
Frequent urination, nervous and irritable, bone demineralization	*Phosphorus:* Found in blueberries, sesame seeds, milk, cheese, fish with small bones
Acne, blemishes, overactive oily skin	*Iodine:* You're getting too much for your system; avoid seafood, iodized salt, spinach, artichokes
Blotchy skin, slow healing, broken veins, white-spotted nails	*Zinc:* Found in shellfish, wheat germ, green leafy vegetables
Brittle nails, weak hair, sagging skin	*Sulfur:* Found in peanuts or peanut butter, clams, beef, lentils, cheese
Cavities, dental problems, wrinkles around the mouth (Good teeth mean better chewing and better digestion—and better skin. Weak teeth cause wrinkles in the mouth area.)	*Fluorine:* Found in fish (especially salt-water fish), tea

Unsaturated Fatty Acids

A dress you make or buy can only be as good as the quality of the fabric; and it is the same with your skin. The quality of your skin depends on many factors: heredity, environment, and life-style. But your skin also depends on what you eat and that is easier for you to control than who your grandparents were.

If you eat a well-balanced, varied selection of foods, you probably are getting all the vitamins you need naturally. But if you diet, you may be low in essential unsaturated fatty acids that are so important to skin health.

Skin grows from the inside out, and the new layers form below the old ones, pushing up on the old ones that are continually shedding off the top. Unsaturated fatty acids are essential to the skin's own maintenance program, as the fatty acids help regulate skin metabolism and monitor the rate of surface-cell shedding. It is available in the following foods:

> lard (and the white fat around meats)
> whole milk
> cereal grains
> vegetable oils such as safflower, corn, olive oil

Because the animal fats are so high in calories compared with the other foods on this list, it might be best to avoid them. But use oil in your salad dressing. Your skin needs them, especially on a stringent reducing diet. A deficiency will make your skin papery and sallow, and in extreme cases, very thin and easily bruised.

How Much Is Enough?

One of the problems with diets is that although most people can remember which foods are forbidden, they never remember that there is no food which can be eaten with impunity—except, perhaps, celery! The average woman of average size with an average-sized stomach can consume about a quart of food at any one time. The term *food* also includes any beverage that you might consume during a two-hour period. Of course a large person, who is in the habit of eating a great deal, might have a stomach of twice that capacity, but that is just what you don't want to be. The stomach, like any internal organ, should not be enlarged abnormally.

If you do overeat and overload your stomach, you will feel uncomfortable, but eventually the stomach stretches to accommodate the food you eat. Your thrifty body will also accommodate your overeating, and store up the excess energy in the form of fat, and you'll find that you're gaining weight.

Remember, a quart is about 4 cups. If you drink a glass of water, and also a cup of coffee or tea, by the time you eat a small sandwich, you will be about full. Most servings in restaurants are ½ to 1 cup in size, and there is more than a quart of servings in even a small meal.

Overeating also has a detrimental effect on the skin. The extra blood that is diverted to the stomach to aid the digestion process is then not available for the skin.

This list of food-intake habits will help you nourish and satisfy your skin *without* overeating.

1. Eat only when you are really hungry. Learn to differentiate between snacking for boredom, anger (yes, biting can be a form of expressing anger that you are unaware of), tension, and other emotions.

2. Chew carefully and slowly. The more you chew, the less you eat. Studies have shown that obese people actually eat much faster than those of normal weight. Chewing food is the first step in digesting it, and better chewing means better digestion, which means more nutrients for building new skin cells. Gulping also confuses your stomach. It takes about 20 minutes for the food to start getting into your bloodstream, and sending messages to your brain to tell you that you are actually satisfied. Fast feasting doesn't give you a chance to know when you are full.

3. Refuse any food that you don't find attractive and satisfying. Learn to refuse foods that you know aren't good for you, and are not useful to your body.

4. See and taste everything you eat. Look at what you are eating and notice the texture, savor the smell, and concentrate on tasting everything carefully. If you do, you'll find that you eat less, but enjoy what you do eat much more. Train yourself to be a food critic.

5. Eat slowly and only when you are in a good mood. Don't dis-

cuss unpleasant news when you're eating, and try to avoid arguments near mealtime.

6. No snacks or absent-minded eating. Every little bit does count.

The Water Diet

All ancient peoples included a water ritual in their festivals and rites, probably because water is the very source of life on earth. Fresh, clear, pure water truly is the only fountain of youth. Water serves three basic health functions.

When you drink water it passes through your throat, moistening the tissues, and then it goes into the stomach. Part of any water you drink is absorbed quickly into your bloodstream through the walls of the stomach. Part of the water goes into your intestines where it helps to keep the food moving swiftly and keeps the food in a liquid stage, helping it to be absorbed through the intestine walls. The watered blood supply is slightly thinned and the thinned blood can speedily distribute foods, nutrients, and oxygen throughout your body.

The fast-flowing blood is constantly moving through every part of the body, and as the water continues to be absorbed, it is also carried into the lymphatic system, where it helps to carry off waste products. There must be an equalization of pressure between the fluids of the lymphatic system and the blood supply in order for the lymphatic process to work, and water helps to keep that delicate balance.

Inside the cells of the skin tissues is a fluid that keeps the cells soft and youthful; that fluid is mostly water. There is a constant exchange between the inside and the outside of the cell walls, and the fluids both inside and outside pass back and forth. Water is essential for all body functions. Absorption, diffusion, and secretion—all are enhanced through the circulation of water.

Water is also needed in the lungs; there can be no intake of oxygen or expulsion of carbon dioxide without it. It soothes the nervous system by lubricating and easing working conditions. If you don't have enough water—even before you are aware you feel thirsty, you might get edgy or irritated. Drinking a glass of water can actually calm your nerves. A drink of fresh water provides the moisture for the delicate neuron cells in your nervous system and in turn those cells promote a sense of well-being.

The sensations of thirst and hunger are frequently confused. Very often you will feel restless or have a gnawing sensation in your stomach; that feeling is not hunger—it is thirst. Before eating always drink. Allow about 20 minutes after you have drunk water to see if the sensation of hunger returns, before choosing a snack or sitting down to a meal.

Water-Fountain Skin-Diet

Morning:	Drink one glass of water as soon as you get up. The water should be cool, but not iced.
Mid-morning:	Drink two glasses of water at about 10 A.M. or two hours after rising, or about two hours before lunch. Try to replace a second cup of coffee with a glass of water.
Lunch:	Drink as much water as you want with your meals. Drinking actually makes the digestion process easier. (Cooks don't like you to drink with meals because it dilutes the strong flavors and seasonings.)
Mid-afternoon:	Two glasses of water. If you are very hungry or feel vaguely unsatisfied, drink tomato juice, or a raw juice pick-up as well. (Don't drink an acid fruit juice such as lemon juice.)
Late-afternoon:	Two glasses of water. If you like to have a late afternoon drink, dilute it with water.
Dinner:	Drink water with dinner; if you drink wine, add water to the wine.
Mid-evening:	Drink two glasses of water about two hours before bedtime.

You can and should drink additional water whenever you think of it, but don't drink more than two 8-ounce glasses at any one time. If you follow a schedule of regular water-drinking, you'll be promoting the process of hydrolysis, the process of chemical decomposition, which is aided by water. This water-wash permits the speedy use of starches, vitamins, sugars, proteins, and other substances for youthful skin and other cell-building functions.

Water also helps in the assimilation of any food you do eat. The first process in the digestive process is preparing the food by chewing and mixing it with saliva. Saliva is almost 99 percent water. The water you drink then carries the food to the stomach where it is broken down and digested with gastric juices, and then carried through the body. The secretions of the stomach wall and the walls of the small intestine contain enzymes that also help to digest the foods. And water is needed to carry all the waste substances through the digestive tract and out of the body. Drinking water is especially important if you eat a high-protein diet.

Under normal conditions the kidneys are one of the main organs of water elimination. The amount of urine produced varies with the water intake. It is usual for one quart of water to carry about one and a half ounces of waste matter dissolved in the urine. A fresh supply of water is essential to keep this process working well. Without the water to carry away the waste, the process of cell growth can suffer or falter.

Which Water and How Much?

Our bodies are two-thirds water, so it is no surprise that water is vital in preventing the dehydration and death of tissues—and skin. It is also vital in maintaining a healthy biochemical activity within the body. We get much of our needed water from the foods we eat, and watery foods such as fruits and vegetables are important in the digestive process. But, perhaps for the first time in history, people now have a chance to choose their drinking water.

Tap water usually comes from ground runoff (lakes, springs, rivers, and streams). Bottled water usually comes from underground sources (wells, underground springs, and rivers), or from captured water such as rainwater.

You can drink distilled water, mineral water, or water that comes from springs or underground rivers. Because the body needs essential minerals, and that supply must be continually replenished, it would seem that mineral water is best. But the body can effectively use only organic minerals. For example, calcium can be used by the body when it is in milk or dairy products; but when it is in the form of dolomite, a calcium clay that is mined as a mineral, it is of no use to the human body. Too many unusable minerals contained in mineral water can be retained by the body and cause health problems, such as kidney stones. Plants, however, *can* convert inorganic minerals into organic minerals; plants growing in iodine-rich soil can be a good source of that mineral for people who need it, or be a problem for salad-lovers who have a tendency to acne.

Rainwater was once thought to be the purest water of all, but unfortunately that is no longer always true. At home, use a water filter if there is any color in your tap water, but make sure to change the filter frequently, because it can become a home for bacteria. For drinking and cosmetic use—such as washing or spraying the face—distilled water is perfect. With distilled water, you won't be consuming inorganic minerals that you cannot use. Also:

- Avoid iced beverages, unless you are dieting (the ice-cold water will temporarily stop hunger pangs)
- Drinking water with greasy food will cause the oils in the foods to solidify—and make them harder to digest.
- Drink with your meals if you wish.
- Don't drink beverages that have been stored in plastic bottles.
- Avoid any drinks with preservatives and acids.
- Drink water slowly; learn to savor its taste.

Eat melons (they are more than 90 percent water) and vegetables to be sure you're getting enough water. And for healthy-looking skin drink at least 10 glasses of water a day—distilled water, if possible, but tap water is actually better for your skin than bottled mineral water.

Water Wizardry

Before enjoying any of these baths, check your tap water to see if it is too alkaline. A quarter of a cup of cider vinegar, or the juice of one small or one-half large lemon, will make your bath skin-soothingly low pH, if you find your water is over a 6.5 pH. To check the water, use Nitrazine (litmus) paper, available at most drugstores, and compare the color of the paper with the color chart on the paper dispenser. Keep your bath water in the "yellow" zone more than the "blue" range.

Hot bath   Invigorating: Water 100°–120°F. Ease into a half-filled tub; soak for about 3 minutes. Turn on cold faucet and gradually cool the bath water. End by splashing or showering in cool water.
Calming: Water 85°–90°F. Ease into a half-filled tub; soak about a minute and gradually add hot water to about 110°F. Remain a minute longer. When you leave this bath, cover your body with avocado or olive oil, wrap up in a sheet, crawl under a blanket, and sleep for about a half hour. (Works well after a tense day.)

Cool bath   Invigorating: Run a cool bath, between 60°–70°F. Sit at the edge of the tub and dangle your legs and feet in the water. When you are comfortable get into tub and splash water on arms, chest, back, and so on. You don't have to be immersed in the water. After a few minutes you'll be recharged.
Calming: Add 1 cup of dried milk to cool bath water. Relax for a few minutes. Then, one at a time, lift your legs up, holding them to the count of 10. Repeat the leg lifts 10 times. The activity will prevent you from getting too cold or bored. Rinse in clean water; you'll find yourself relaxed.

One of the rules of water therapy is not to remain in a hot tub for very long. It can wash away your body oils, and it can weaken the tissue. Never allow your chest to soak under warm water. The weight of the breast will encourage stretching of the thin, muscle-free breast tissue. Keep your baths no longer than 10 minutes to protect your skin.

Never put oil on your skin before you bathe; apply it mid-bath. The oil will act as a barrier, preventing the water from cleaning and moistening your skin. After about 5 to 8 minutes in the bath, apply oil to your skin, coating it lightly. The oil will then hold in the coating of moisture and protect the plumped-up, waterlogged skin cells.

Water Wizardry (cont'd)

When you soak in a warm bath, you're increasing the blood supply to the skin's surface and to the surface muscles. Pulsating water also increases blood circulation, and this can stimulate new skin growth. But remember, your skin is softer and more vulnerable when it is wet and moist. You can bruise easily, and fast changes in skin temperature can encourage broken surface veins—those tiny lines that will not go away. Treat wet skin with tenderness.

Water Massage

Water is nature's best beauty aid for the face. The French are well aware of the benefits of hydrotherapy, and they have created several devices for applying water to various parts of the body to keep them taut and smooth. Clarins, the French cosmetic company, got started as a beauty salon and their special feature was the use of water as a treatment for the breasts, arms, inner thighs, and other parts of the body and the face. They are devoted to the beneficial effects of cold water on tissue, and believe that cold water will tighten and tone almost all skin tissue.

The French technique is to aim a specially designed cup at the skin. A cold water supply is attached to the cup and a fine strong spray of icy water is bulleted on the skin. This has a stimulating effect on the skin, and causes the muscles and skin to tighten and hold. You can get a similar effect if you aim a fine spray of icy water from a shampoo spray at your chest. The breasts will immediately tighten and firm, and the effect will last for several hours.

Here is how you can make your own hydrotherapy mask at home. You'll need a hose with a shower head or shampoo fixture. They are available in most drugstores and in some hardware stores. You'll also need a shower cap that is very heavy duty, or a real rubber bathing cap. Attach the bathing cap to the hose so that the shower head is inside the cap. You'll probably have to make a small hole in the cap so that the cold water can spray out of the hose through the tiny nozzle openings in the head, and onto your face. Hold the cap tightly against the sides of your face, but not so tightly that you cut out all the air—you need to breathe.

Pin your hair back or cover it with another shower cap. Turn on the cold water from your basin water tap. Hold the cap against your face so that the water showers your face and not your bathroom, and enjoy the prickling and tingling sensation of cold water shooting at your skin. Don't put the pressure on too strongly—you don't want to bruise your skin, just invigorate it.

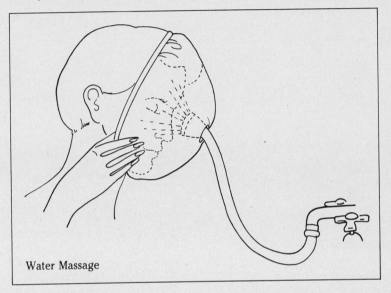

Water Massage

Skin-Savers

From time to time wonder treatments, new revolutionary products, and miracle devices for better skin appear on the market. They usually work—a little bit. They work to some extent because each of them depends on some tried and true method of skin care, but approaches it in a new way. The following are six popular wrinkle-fighting ideas. There are books devoted to each of them, but the essence of each technique or method is one of the basic approaches to skin care. Remember, your skin is unique, so try them all, but use only those routines that are most pleasant for you and give you the best results.

Facial Exercises for Firm, Tight Skin

Exercise benefits skin tone and texture because it dilates the vascular system and brings an increased supply of blood, oxygen, and nutrients to the skin. Exercises for the face expand and contract the facial muscles—this stimulates the nerves of the face, and helps to relax cramped muscles and soothe jangled nerves.

Some people are more muscular than others, and many find that facial exercises really work!

Before doing any of these exercises, cover your face and throat with a heavy coat of vegetable oil. Keep warm: You don't want your muscles to cramp or your skin to tighten.

Facial Exercises Everyone Can Do

These will help tone up facial muscles and skin, and help you relax, too.

1. *To soothe puffiness and firm up eyelids:* Open eyes wide and stare, then squeeze them tightly shut. Repeat several times.

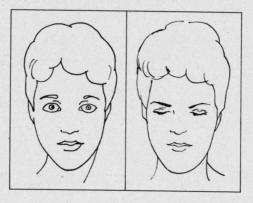

2. *To discourage forehead lines and stimulate scalp muscles:* Hold head still and look straight ahead. Raise eyebrows and forehead skin as high as you can. Feel the movement of the scalp and muscles around the ears. Relax. Repeat energetically several times.

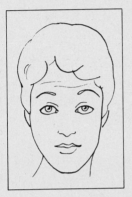

3. *To discourage lines around the mouth:* Force an exaggerated smile with mouth closed. Then relax lips. Pucker up lips as far as possible, then relax. With mouth shut, puff out cheeks, and blow air from side to side several times. Then slowly blow air out. Repeat each exercise.

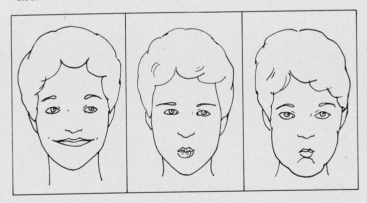

4. *To firm up chin line:* Open mouth as wide as possible. Thrusting lower lip out and up, try to touch nose. Repeat several times.

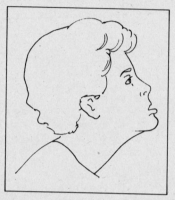

5. *To firm neck muscles and discourage wrinkles,* repeat the following exercises several times:
— Throw head back. Jut chin and lower lip forward. Relax.
— Stick out tongue. Stretch it up to touch tip of nose. Relax.
— Sit at table. Place elbow on table and make fist under chin. Push down on fist with chin, at the same time, try to lift head upward with fist. (Elbow must remain on table.) Relax.

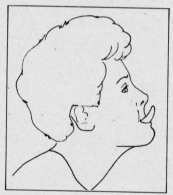

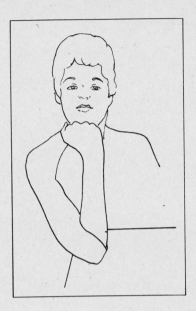

Collagen

The lower level of skin, the dermis is the home of the blood vessels, nerves, and glands that supply the skin, and also of fibroelastic connective tissue that gives the skin its ability to return to its shape when it is moved, or pinched. This connective tissue contains two types of elastic fibers: collagen and elastin. They are both important parts of normal youthful skin—and when they are weakened the skin looks older.

Collagen is a recent "wonder" ingredient in many skin creams and treatments and many of the leaders of the cosmetics industry are touting the miraculous de-aging effect collagen creams can have on older skin. Cosmetic collagen, a protein, comes from cattle skin. Under the microscope, the collagen fibers are almost identical to the structure of human connective tissue. But spending $25 or more on a collagen cream is not spending your money wisely; you can get the same results with most moisturizers, at a much lower price.

Collagen applied directly to the skin does not produce spectacular results, nor can it permanently remove wrinkles or restore the skin's elasticity, for the molecular structure of the collagen does not permit it to be absorbed through the skin.

However, collagen in liquid form *can* be a real rejuvenator when it is injected into the skin. A liquid collagen (Zyderm) is now used for implants, which are a safe and effective means of treating areas of the face previously not amenable to other correction. These areas include depressed scars, fine forehead and smile lines, furrows between the brows, acne scars, and other areas not sufficiently affected by a face-lift.

Liquid collagen is assimilated by the body, once it has been injected, and the implant becomes the same consistency as normal skin tissue. When test biopsies were performed during the experimental stages of developing liquid collagen for implants and wrinkle erasure, it was noticed that the collagen soon was actually identical to the recipient's own tissues. Dr. Steven Herman, a pioneer in the use of cosmetic collagen injections, describes how liquid collagen works:

> The collagen is implanted by your physician into your skin. This is done by injecting the collagen with a very fine needle. The injection is made right at the depression or scar or wrinkle. The loss of original tissue in the area was the source of the wrinkle; it allowed the skin to loosen. So, the collagen implant acts as a replacement for that lost tissue. The implant fills in the depression and raises the skin surface to the level of the surrounding tissue. The wrinkle, or scar, then seems to vanish.

Collagen in liquid form, used in the skin, can only be injected by a doctor and should not be confused with collagen in creams that can be bought over the counter. Before undergoing liquid collagen treatment, prospective patients must be tested for any sort of negative reaction they might have to the substance. This is done by injecting a small amount into the forearm. If after one month's time there is no abnormal reaction, the collagen treatment can begin.

If you've been using a collagen cream and you've actually noticed some positive effects, such as the plumping of the skin, be assured it is *not* because the collagen has been absorbed by your skin. This plumping results from collagen's hydrophilic properties; like many other ingredients in many other skin creams, collagen attracts water from the air. The same effect may be achieved using other, less-expensive proteins commonly found in inexpensive creams and moisturizers, or in home-created products.

If you're still curious about the effects of topical collagen, here are natural, inexpensive recipes for three different facial masks based on natural protein substances: egg, beef, and chicken.

EGG COLLAGEN MASK

1 egg yolk, well beaten

Rinse face with warm water. Do not dry. Apply the yolk of a beaten egg to the face with a basting brush or your fingers, and cover face with a moist warm towel. Relax for about 15 minutes. Remove the towel, and rinse the face and the towel in cool water. Be sure to rinse thoroughly; the heat from the towel and the skin's natural warmth will cause the egg to become harder and sticky.

*Egg yolks contain a great deal of sulfur and so it is excellent when used as a wash to heal acne.

BEEF COLLAGEN MASK

¼ beef patty, raw

Close your eyes and apply ¼ of the beef patty to the skin around each eye. Relax for 10 minutes. Wash away the residue with warm water. The beef's cooling, calming effect is the reason behind the folk remedying of soothing a black eye with a raw steak.

CHICKEN COLLAGEN MASK

The next time you buy chicken breasts or thighs, try this:

5 small pieces of chicken skin

As you peel the skin from the chicken, notice the inside of the skin. It is covered with a slimy mucous membrane. It is this membrane that makes chicken skin an excellent mask. Lie down and arrange the chicken skin over the eyes, mouth, and forehead. Allow the skin to remain on your face for about 10 minutes. Wash the residue away with cool water.

These masks do not penetrate the skin, but they all contain heavy concentrations of collagen, and they all will block evaporation of your skin's natural moisture.

Hormone Creams

Some skin creams include estrogen, a female hormone, in their formula. There is a theory that the hormones somehow counteract weaknesses in the skin caused by lower hormone levels associated with aging.

The dermis, or second layer of the skin, of an older person is usually thinner than that of a young person. The creams that contain hormones can help the skin to retain more water (moisture) and so to be thicker, plumper, and seem more youthful. The other ingredients in the creams contain a fat covering for the skin, and it is questionable if it is the oil in the creams, or the hormones, that bring results. Most doctors think it is the oil that acts as a barrier. Creams with hormones are very expensive, because the price of chemically produced hormones is far higher than that of an oil.

Some special cell-repair creams claim to help the cells in the dermis repair themselves so that they can retain moisture for longer periods of time. If the dermis could be made to hold enough water, it would provide a soft, full, strong support for the skin, the small wrinkles of the skin would be smoothed out, and the skin would look softer and more elastic. There seems to be very little evidence, however, that any cream can actually help the cells repair themselves. New cells are constantly growing to replace dead and worn cells, but the cells don't seem to be able to mend themselves once they cease to hold moisture, dry out, and die.

Urea

In ancient times, Babylonian women kept their skin soft and supple by wrapping themselves in urine-soaked cloths. Later beauties, including the Egyptians, also used urine for skin and hair treatments.

If you want to take advantage of the benefits of urea in a more sanitary and acceptable manner, there are skin-care products containing chemically created urea on the market. Aquacare/HP Lotion (Herbert) is one of the best. It is available in both 3 percent urea and 10 percent solutions. Check the labels on other cosmetics; urea cosmetics can make the skin soft, smooth, and clear without clogging the pores.

Vitamin A Acid Treatments for Aging

Vitamin A acid treatments have been used for acne for several years, and now they are also thought to be of potential use in slowing the aging of the skin. Dr. Albert Kligman, a noted professor of dermatology at the University of Pennsylvania School of Medicine and one of the leading researchers in skin aging, confirmed in an interview with *Prevention* magazine that although very little is known of exactly how the vitamin A acid works, it does increase blood flow. Increased blood flow stimulates the skin and the skin then lays down a little bit more of the gelatinlike substance that keeps it supple. Dr. Kligman added, "It helps with aging skin. You take someone who is 40, and whose skin isn't showing too much sign of age, and who is committed to sunscreens and greases—vitamin A acid will help her."

Interest in vitamin A acid began in the 1930s when it was noticed that a deficiency of this vitamin caused the skin's surface to thicken, become rough, and the pores to clog easily, mostly because of the thickening and clogging of the epidermal cells. Doctors theorized that if too little vitamin A could cause thickening of the upper layer, one of the sign's of aging, perhaps an excess supply would cause the opposite—a thinning. The problem was that high dosages of vitamin A, taken internally, can be damaging to the liver. It was in the early 1960s that Dr. Kligman and his staff at the University of Pennsylvania applied an acid of vitamin A directly to the skin, and discovered that external treatment with vitamin A does thin the skin, with no danger to the liver.

Vitamin A acid seems to speed up the formation, maturing, flattening, and dying of skin cells. The result is that the life of the cells is shorter, and the skin cells are renewed more quickly. With vitamin A, the flattening or keratinization of the cells is so fast that the old cells don't clump together, and the epidermis doesn't become tough, thick, or coarse. The vitamin A acid also affects the cells within the hair follicles, where they have a tendency to pack in the shrunken older pores. (It is clumped, densely packed cells more than the oil that clog the pores and cause blackheads and whiteheads.) Vitamin A acid acts to make the upper cells form loosely and flake off easily.

The little wrinkles of the skin will flatten out when they are treated with a vitamin A acid peel, with the result that the entire skin will show increased healing power. The full-strength acid can be bought only with a prescription, although it is also found in diluted levels in some cosmetics. Lactic acid, rich in vitamin A, also can be used as a vitamin A skin-thinner.

Because peeling with vitamin A can result in peeling and thinning of the upper layer of skin, the skin is more vulnerable to irritants, to sunburn, and to evaporation of moisture. Harsh astringents or alkaline soaps can also damage the skin's fresh new cells very easily.

Many dermatologists use vitamin A acid for acne because it does encourage peeling, and that helps to clear the skin of blemishes by keeping the pores open. Vitamin A acid is one of the most potent substances in skin care, and it is a real rejuvenator, but you should consult your doctor or dermatologist if you would like to learn more about its uses.

Plastic-Wrap Your Skin for a Glowing Complexion

You can use ordinary kitchen plastic wrap to encourage the action of spot skin treatments. The wrap, although lethal if you put it over your head with no allowance for breathing, can be used to keep soothing unguents or cosmetic masks on the skin for short periods of time. *Never use a wrap for more than 15 minutes.* An added plus is that there is a slight irritation from covering the skin with a wrap, and that irritation makes the skin soften and fill, providing a temporary smoothing-out of small lines. Many dancers, models, and actresses use the following "tricks" to multiply any treatment's effects.

An additional word of caution: Although most of the skin's oxygen is supplied by the bloodstream, the skin does play a small role in absorbing oxygen and eliminating carbon dioxide and waste gases directly from the air. Not allowing that carbon dioxide to leave the cells can cause eventual cell damage; carbon dioxide is toxic. Blocking the natural perspiration of the body is also counter to the best health of anyone with diabetes, high blood pressure, or heart problems.

For the Face: Covering the cheeks and forehead with a light wrapping of plastic over a nutrient-rich mask slows the drying of the mask, and will encourage the soothing and lubricating action of any mask. You can easily do this by cutting a hole for your nose in a sheet of plastic wrap, and draping the wrap over your face, with only the nose out in the air. Don't tighten the plastic; it should just lightly cover your mask.

For the Neck: Pin your hair up or cover with a shower cap. Coat your neck and shoulders with a rich mask or oil. Wrap your neck and shoulders with about 18 inches of plastic wrap.

For the Feet: Using plastic vegetable bags, you can cover your feet with oil, and then place them in the plastic bags. Tie the ends together to hold the bag securely, and allow your feet, inside the bags, to sit in a warm tub of water. The warm water will keep the oil warm, and the bags will prevent the oil from floating all over the tub and being lost. In about 10 minutes your feet will be refreshed and smoothed. Rinse your feet in cool water, but do not cool too rapidly, because that will injure the small blood vessels near the surface of your skin.

For the Hands: Using sandwich bags, cut four small slots in the bottom of each bag for your fingers. Coat the backs of the hands with vegetable oil, and then slide the hand into the bag so that the fingers protrude through the slits, and if it is comfortable, make a small slit on the side for your thumb. Wear these hand-mitts when you're cleaning and working around the house. You'll be getting a beauty treatment, and your fingers will be free for action.

If you wrap up the entire hand, this method will do a good job of readying your hands for a manicure—the oil will cleanse and soften your nails.

Knees and Legs: An all-over treatment is wonderful for dry, scaly legs, especially during those long, steam-heated winters. Slough off the chapped or dry sections, then coat with cream or oil and wrap the legs (this works for arms, too) in plastic wrap. Remember—no more than 10 or 12 minutes for this treatment—it's not wise to keep such large areas of skin covered for too long.

If you want to tighten the softening thighs, and perhaps reduce a cellulite deposit, rub a mixture of ivy extract on the thighs before wrapping them. Ivy extract can be obtained at some health food stores. A 10-minute treatment at home will temporarily firm up the skin—but it will not have a long-lasting effect on the cellulite; only loss of weight can accomplish that.

Love Is the Skin's Best Friend

You've probably noticed that you look better when you're in love; and you may have observed others in love and noticed how they seem suddenly more graceful, healthy, and their skin seems to glow.

Sexual love is perhaps the best therapy for skin beauty. Sexual excitement makes the organs expand as blood accumulates in the pelvic region. The breasts and the nipples also respond, and become engorged with blood. The heart, which usually beats at the rate of 72 times a minute, speeds up, and it might beat twice or three times its normal rate. The blood rushes to the skin's surface, and there is a blush of color over the face, neck, and chest. That supply of blood refreshes, cleanses, and builds the skin. It makes the skin thicker, denser.

During sexual arousal your breath, and the oxygen that it carries, also change. Breathing goes from the normal of about 20 breaths a minute to about twice that number. The invigorating supply of oxygen and blood will return to normal after orgasm.

When you are in love, and make love fully and often, you'll probably look your most beautiful. Your complexion will appear more youthful, and your muscle tone will be much better: even your nails grow longer and stronger, and your hair will become shinier and thicker. You may even notice some changes around your eyes. During foreplay the iris of the eyes enlarge, and during the orgasm stage they contract. The activity of the pupils exercises all of the round muscles that hold your eyeball in place, and the movement can smooth out the small lines on the outer eye and keep the eyeballs smooth, clear, and bright.

During lovemaking the facial muscles firm noticeably: The furrows that run from the nose to the outer corners of the mouth fill in, and the cheeks become plumper. Because the muscles tighten the little pouches on the lower jowls and near the mouth disappear, and the neck becomes much more flexible because the muscles of the shoulders and the back of the neck are completely relaxed.

There is lots of good news about the beauty effects of sex for you, but the rumor that sex is a substitute for a basic exercise program is ill-founded. If you really go at it for about an hour you can burn off from 250 to 450 calories, but that isn't anywhere near what a good aerobics class can do.

If at present you don't have a lover who you find truly exciting, all is not lost. With a little imagination, and some concentration on your own personal fantasies, you can create some excitement. Sexy thoughts lead to a better love life and a smoother skin.

Stop Giving Yourself Wrinkles

The quasi-science of phrenology was popular in Victorian times. The theory was that character could be read through feeling the bumps on the head and scalp. Another popular theory was that certain proportions for facial features could be used to identify personality and intelligence. Both of these theories have been discredited, but the old belief that you look more like yourself as you get older may have some basis in fact. An internationally known surgeon believes that the way wrinkles form gives evidence of your facial habits and patterns of thought. For example, people with lines between their eyes are intense and careful; people with wrinkles over their brows are skeptical and not easily fooled; pursing the lips shows a tight, distrustful personality. Perhaps this theory isn't any better than the others—but people do cling to them, and why let people respond to your wrinkles rather than the real you! Here is a simple, inexpensive way to use behavior modification on yourself and rid yourself of wrinkle-inducing facial habits.

Buy 100 one-cent stamps at the nearest post office. (The regular stamps work well, but the commemorative stamps are really best because they are larger, and seem to have a stronger glue backing. They are prettier, too.) Moisten the glued backing slightly with water and paste the stamp over any wrinkle. You might have to hold the skin smooth with the fingers of one hand while you're applying the stamp with the other to make sure you're not pasting over a wrinkle. The stamp will remind you not to move your face in any way that would crinkle the stamp, and will help you stop any habitual grimace.

The stamp or stamps (depending on the length of the wrinkle) will also temporarily smooth out the skin. Covering the skin prevents evaporation from the skin's surface, and it also irritates the skin slightly. The body responds to that minor irritation by sending blood and fluids to the surface of the skin to protect it. This blood rush plumps out the skin and makes the wrinkle vanish—temporarily.

Some skin-care experts recommend taping the skin with surgical tape. The tape has the same effect as the stamps—it reminds you not to grimace, and helps you break any facial expression habits as well as causing mild skin irritation. Tape does more harm than good, however, because peeling or tearing the tape from the skin pulls at delicate skin, and can damage connective tissue. Another problem is that tape leaves a gummy residue on the skin.

Stamps are easily removed with just plain water, and leave no residue that must be washed away with strong chemicals. If you buy 100 one-cent stamps, you should find that by the time you've used about 60 cents worth, the wrinkle-making habits should be modified, and your face will be smoother and less tense-looking.

4

Know Your Skin's Enemies

Skin Changes You Can Reverse

There are continual changes in your skin, happily some of the worst are only temporary. Some days, for unknown reasons, your skin might look older, and even more wrinkled. Then, after a night's sleep, a vacation, or a change in diet your skin can bounce back. Temporary changes in the skin are not significant.

Temporary changes usually vanish spontaneously, or can be treated and corrected. For example, a rash brought on by an allergy will vanish as soon as the fabric or plant or offensive substance is removed. And, to speed allergy treatment, antihistamines can bring almost instant relief.

The change in the acid/alkaline balance of the skin due to emotions, or because of the menstrual cycle, or pregnancy, can invite temporary blemishes. During this time the skin becomes slightly more oily, and slightly more alkaline. This leads to thickening of the epidermis and clogging of the pores with bacteria-attracting dead skin cells.

Chapping, sunburn, and allergic reactions to detergents can all cause temporary peeling. A rapid loss of the horny layer is brought on by the drying and death of skin cells. By tanning, the skin tries to defend itself, and it darkens in just a few hours in an attempt to block the rays of sun from the delicate under layers. Dehydration causes the upper layer of the skin to flake off, as the tanning process continues. Tanning is a temporary change in skin color.

Unfortunately, there are permanent changes, too. Permanent changes in the skin are different because they are usually caused by some internal modification within the body, or within the structure of the skin itself. Sometimes when a temporary condition (such as irritating the skin with an allergy-producing substance) continues, it can eventually cause a basic skin change.

Sun damage can be an example of permanent change, too. First there is a temporary change in the surface and some temporary change in the color. But years later, after repeated exposure to the harmful ultraviolet rays, the internal basic change is evidenced in an obvious weakening of the connective tissue. Smoking can also make permanent changes in the skin by affecting the way the oxygen is used by the cells.

The skin on your face right now can probably provide you with examples of both temporary and permanent changes. Some of the signs of age on your face are permanent, but some are only temporary. The first step in skin care is to know your own skin, and realize that some areas of the skin are naturally very different from other areas and you must treat each section in a different way.

Here is a list of most common temporary and permanent complexion problems:

Acne (temporary). Blemishes and surface infections will appear in areas of the skin where the sebum production is abnormally high and the elimination of waste products and skin cells is abnormally low. Decreased production of the skin's oil glands is natural as you age. Thorough washing and exfoliating can bring fast improvement. The scars caused by pimples can be permanent, which is why treatment is always necessary.

Coarse, oily skin (temporary). This condition is marked by leathery skin with large pores and a dull, sallow skin-tone. Immediate improvement can be made by thinning the epidermis through exfoliation. Clean pores appear smaller, and the irritation of the abrasion makes them temporarily smaller still. The texture of the skin is improved by stimulating a vigorous blood supply.

Dry, dehydrated skin (temporary). When there is insufficient oil production from the oil glands, the surface of the skin dries out easily, and the texture becomes rough. You cannot make your oil glands produce more than your age and genetic makeup allow—but you can use a light vegetable oil as a replacement for your own natural oils.

Flaky, rough skin (temporary). When the skin is very dry or irritated, the horny layer thickens and then sloughs off in clumps. Rid the surface of your skin of these flakes by exfoliation. The texture of your skin will improve and your skin will feel more comfortable (the dry flakes often are itchy).

Blotchy or red skin (sometimes permanent). When the dermis layer thins, the blood vessels are closer to the surface, where they are less protected and less insulated from temperature changes and bruises. Those vulnerable blood vessels can dilate and rupture from heat or undue pressure, giving the skin a "road map" appearance. The capillaries in the skin are very thin and fragile, and a blotchy skin can indicate a permanent breakdown in the system. Reduce the chance of any further damage by avoiding extremes in temperature and rough treatment. Broken blood vessels can be treated by a dermatologist.

Aged skin (permanent). Youthful wrinkles from dehydration are different from the problems of aged skin. Age makes the collagen and elastic fibers that bind the skin weak and thin and less elastic. With age, connective tissue breaks and the entire surface of the skin becomes covered with wrinkles, streaks, and sags. You can avoid weakening the collagen by avoiding anything that pulls at the skin or moves the skin from the underlying tissues. Depriving your skin of water, oxygen, and nutrients such as protein speeds the collapse of the collagen. New techniques in cosmetic surgery can excise aging skin and reinforce natural collagen.

Liver spots (permanent). These flat brown spots appear on the hands, forehead, and sides of the face. They are encouraged by sunlight, and usually appear on dry and aged skin. Vitamin A acid shows great promise in treating age-spots.

Do You Recognize Your Own Skin?

Professionals in skin care learn to recognize the symptoms of dry, oily, or combination skin only after months of training, and many people have sensitive or dehydrated skin without even realizing it. The fact that 90 percent of all adults have both dry and oily areas of skin complicates skin care; it is like trying to wear comfortable clothes when your right side will be in summer and your left will be in winter—and you're allergic to wool! Here are some clues to finding your skin type:

Oily skin: A shiny surface, enlarged pores, whiteheads, and blackheads on most areas of your face, and even on your shoulders, indicate an oily skin.

Dry skin: A rough or coarse surface that appears poreless is typical of dry skin. There may be small lines around your eyes and mouth. Your skin is tight after washing.

Combination skin: Your nose, forehead, and chin are oily, but your cheeks, throat, and eyes are dry. You're never sure what product to use because you don't want to add oil to one part or dry out another.

Sensitive skin: If your skin often feels itchy, or turns red or becomes blotchy, you may have sensitive skin. Your skin can be sensitive to pollen, weather changes, alcohol, coffee, stress—and several hundred other situations or products. You'll have to take extra care of your skin—all your life.

Dehydrated skin: If your skin's cells do not retain an adequate amount of moisture, your skin becomes dehydrated. It will flake, crack, and look papery and probably be covered with fine lines. Your skin's natural oils usually block the evaporation of the skin's moisture, but you can be oily and dehydrated at the same time. Drinking at least 10 glasses of water a day can help, and so can living in a very moist climate.

Your Skin's Worst Enemy

The skin's most dangerous enemy feels warm and looks cheerful. Although a suntan gives the illusion of health and vitality, in 15 to 20 years the cumulative effects of the sun's rays will cause wrinkling, aging, irregular texture, and uneven color.

Dr. Jim Baral, director of the New York Dermatology Center, affiliated with Mt. Sinai Hospital, suggests limiting outdoor activities during the spring and summer months to before 10 A.M. and after 4 P.M. Dr. Baral also recommends the use of sunscreens containing PABA, because they tend to combine with the skin. If you apply a sun-block lotion once or twice a day for about a week *before* going out in the sun, the skin will build up a tolerance level for sun exposure. You might consider a sun-block lotion as a basic summertime grooming aid.

Jim Baral has another suggestion for those especially sensitive to the burning effects of the sun's rays. There is some evidence that taking two aspirins before exposure to the sun, and following up with two aspirins every 6 hours for the next 24 to 36 hours, can lessen the harsh effects of the sun's rays. However, Baral warns that this aspirin regime is not suitable for anyone with allergies, or where there has been any contraindication for aspirin; he further advises checking with your own physician before taking the aspirins.

Sun Protection

A comprehensive program of protection can help to prevent the aging effects of the sun on the skin without resigning yourself to the life of a mole. The right program can also shelter the skin from the injurious "physical" and "chemical" elements—including friction from wind and water, dehydration from wind and water, irritating acidic or alkaline pollutants in the atmosphere, and salt, copper and chlorine in the water, if you swim.

Of all the attacks on your skin, the most destructive ones are the subtle ultraviolet rays that shrink and harden the elastic collagen in the dermis, below the surface of your skin. This causes the skin to lose its elasticity and resiliency. The shrinkage that occurs with the sun exposure was, until recently, thought to be irreversible. The effects are known to be cumulative, and each exposure can add lines and wrinkles to your face; but now there is some hope. Dr. Albert Kligman, professor of Dermatology at the University of Pennsylvania School of Medicine, has noted that studies with animals show that when the sun exposure is stopped, there is some evidence that the tissue can regenerate to a more normal state, the thick irregular outer layer that was damaged by the sun thins somewhat, and the little growths, freckles, and blotches seem to modify slightly. What this means for the average woman is that even if you've been in the sun too often, and stayed too long, your skin can improve—slowly, but it can happen.

Don't depend on possible skin recovery, however: without protection the sun can do real damage now. To prevent that damage, use moisturizers, foundations, lipsticks, and even protective eye products with built-in sun guards. Most dermatologists now recommend a sunscreen with a SPF (Sun Protective Factor) of at least 15, or maximum protection. The degree of protection is determined by a standard government test that measures the ability or inability of the skin to withstand the sun without burning between the hours of 11 A.M. and 3 P.M. But you must consider the following factors:

— Certain medications (birth control pills, blood pressure medicine, etc.) can affect the skin's reaction to the sun.
— Altitude is important. If you live on top of a mountain many more of the sun's rays can penetrate easily through the clear, thin air.
— Reflective surfaces such as snow or sand can mean you need more protection than if you were on grass.
— Atmospheric conditions and wind make a difference, and you can damage your skin without ever feeling hot or turning red. You *can* get a sunburn on a hazy day.
— Seasonal differences in the sun's rays make a big difference, and the strength of the rays near the equator is greater than farther north.

Use sun protection continuously—from the first time you go out in the sun to the last. Don't be deceived into thinking that a slight tanning of the skin will provide any protection. It takes at least two days for melanin, a chemical produced by the skin as a protection against the sun's ultraviolet rays, to give you some protective skin coloring; and even a warm, brown, even tan does not provide complete blockage from the sun's rays.

Always select an outdoor protection that consists of two qualities: look for a Sun Protective Factor (SPF) of at least 15, or the words "ultra" sunscreen, and a cream that will moisturize and protect against the harsh drying effects of the outdoors. A good SPF 15 cream will let you stay in the sun 15 times longer without burning than you could without it. Dr. Diana Bihova, a New York dermatologist, stresses that the applying sunscreen one or two hours before going out in the sun can enhance the action of the screen. She also advises the use of lip protectors that have a sunscreen. A sunscreen gloss guards the lips from the sun's ultraviolet rays and the emollient in the gloss keeps the lips from drying and helps them stay soft and moist. Look for a lip screen that also has a high protective number.

Even Skin Tone

There are many different types of color problems that affect your skin. One of the most common is excessive and uneven skin pigmentation. When one area of the skin is darker in color than your usual skin tone, or when there is a dense profusion of dark spots on the skin's surface, it can ruin your looks. The dark spots are usually freckles, chloasma—"liver spots," or flat moles. Skin bleaches may remedy some of these pigmentation problems.

Bleaching creams have been used for centuries. When farming was the major occupation of the masses, a pale complexion was much sought after as a sign of status. Most of the ancient formulas for bleaching the skin used mercury, or mercury compounds, and were quite effective. In 1974 the Federal Food and Drug Administration banned the use of any bleach cream with mercury, which is potentially toxic, and can cause degeneration of the human nervous system.

Since the prohibition of the use of mercury, commercial skin bleaches usually rely on hydroquinone as the active bleaching agent. Hydroquinone creams can, after six to eight weeks of application, decrease the amount of pigment in the skin. But the creams are not suitable for large areas. The hydroquinone creams cannot bleach normal skin to a lighter tone; they can only restore hyperpigmented skin to its original, or close to original, shade. The use of bleach creams is a long process. During the time that you use a cream you should avoid any exposure to the sun. One way of speeding the effects of a hydroquinone bleach cream is to mix it with crushed aspirins (salicylic acid) which will peel old skin and make the bleach more effective.

There are occasional irritations from the application of some bleaches, and especially bleaches that rely on lemon as a bleaching agent have been known to cause skin irritations.

Dark-skinned people seem more vulnerable to pigmentation problems than naturally light-complexioned people; inflammatory skin disease can produce dark, gray, or even blue-black patches.

Chloasma is also called the mask of pregnancy. It is one of the skin-color irregularities that most often affects young women. It is common in pregnant women, and also in women who are taking birth-control pills. Sometimes the brownish darkening around the upper cheeks and forehead fades naturally, but often it responds only to a bleach. The first sign of this darkening, usually in your twenties, means that you have a tendency to discoloration. Once you know you have that tendency, you'll have to be ever watchful against situations that can bring on discolorations. (See also page 87 for chemical substances that can cause allergic reactions.)

Why Scars Are Formed

When skin is damaged, and the damage goes below the epidermis level into the dermis level, there is always a chance that when it heals there may be an area of smooth, hairless, inelastic skin, marking where the skin was damaged. This skin is scar tissue. The skin can regenerate itself only if enough of the germinative layer of the epidermis is left for it to slowly and continually replenish itself. When the damage goes below the epidermis line and destroys the area of germination, which is deepest in the area around the hair follicle, then it is impossible for the skin to reproduce itself, and a scar is formed. That is the reason why scar tissue doesn't have hair follicles.

Keloids are scar tumors that do *not* become malignant. They do, however, grow larger than the original area of damage. Keloids are harmless, although unattractive. Burns have more of a tendency to produce keloid tissue than do cuts or other wounds. Blacks develop keloid scars ten times more often than do whites. Black women should be very careful about any damage to their skin—especially piercing the ears. The piercing can cause keloids to grow around the pierced skin of the earlobe, which makes wearing any earrings very uncomfortable.

Steroid injections have been used to diminish scar tissue, and recently, collagen in liquid form has been used to pump up and level off depressed scars and small "ice-pick" holes that can result from severe acne.

Stretch marks are not a form of scarring although they may be similar in appearance. Many experts claim there is little that can be done to erase these light-colored tracks that mark the tummy, lower abdomen, thighs, buttocks, or other parts of the body, but they can be made less noticeable by bleaching the surrounding skin.

Stretch marks are technically called *striae,* meaning channels or furrows in Latin. They are usually seen after the skin has been distended, beyond its flexibility. When this happens the underlying elastic proteins of the skin break down, and the epidermis and dermis become detached from the fibrous collagen tissue. Stretch marks are a form of damage to the skin but do no real harm.

Surgery can eliminate some of the marks, because you are eliminating some of the skin. But for most, a soothing bleach cream mixed with vitamin E will substantially lighten the area around the stretch mark so it is less noticeable.

The Birth of the Blemish

Because of continual skin cell growth the pores often get clogged with dead cells that clump together and form bumps under the surface of the skin. These bumps become whiteheads or blackheads. When oil, skin cells, and other material cannot make their way out of blocked pores, or makeup clogs the pore openings from the surface, then the waste materials force their way through the walls of the tiny pores. When the walls break down, bacteria become a problem and there is usually an infection. That small infection is a blemish; a red, tender, and ugly area.

Warmth or steaming the skin dilates the surface pore openings, and brings blood to the surface of the skin, so the waste-disposal system of the body can carry off some of the old cells. But the best way to keep the skin blemish-free is to periodically wisk away some of the dead cells that form the top layer of skin. This opens the pores, and allows the oils, dead cells from inside the pore walls, and other waste matter to move upward and outward to the surface of the skin. The heat also has a tendency to stimulate oil glands, so after allowing your skin to cool naturally, rinse it with cold water to slow oil-gland action.

Emotional Skin

Do you blush in embarrassment; or pale with fear; or redden with anger? These are all signs of how your emotions affect your skin. Skin is a mirror of your psychic reactions–from great happiness to great pain. Stress can make your skin itch, burn, and perspire with no apparent exterior cause; it can produce a florid rash, or a display of hives, pustules, or blisters. Repressed emotions can also produce a sallow, deadly ashen color.

Adult forms of acne often occur during times of stress or directly after a stressful period. The French connect the skin disorder psoriasis with emotions, and many medical experts believe hair loss in women is stress-induced.

Acne rosacea, sometimes mistakenly confused with acne, is a reddening and swelling of some areas of the face; particularly the nose, and is sometimes described as a "blush gone wrong." It is more common among women than men, but W. C. Fields, who was a victim, is often associated with the disorder because of his huge misshapen nose. Rosacea begins with a flushing in the affected area; after a time the flushing becomes permanent; it doesn't subside. The skin in the area thickens and eventually eruptions appear. The nose or other affected area becomes enlarged.

High-powered, driven women—especially women who are fair—are vulnerable to this condition. When it strikes, nose, chin, cheeks, and the forehead where it appears are covered with pimples and tiny broken blood vessels that leave the skin angry and reddened. Dr. Peter N. Horvath, a Washington D.C. dermatologist, believes the problem is that the blush mechanism becomes exhausted, and can no longer regulate itself. Strong feelings, alcohol, hot drinks, spicy food, and other stimulants can cause or exacerbate the condition. If you have a tendency toward this condition, and your face is flushed and often angry-looking, you should be very cautious about any further stimulation to your skin. Rather than exfoliating your skin with a strong abrasive or a chemical that will whisk away the surface dead cells, you should be concerned about guarding your delicate complexion from any further excitement.

Rosacea responds to antibiotics, reports Dr. Horvath. "We don't know why they work, but they do." Along with medication, he advises avoiding hard liquor and spicy foods. Cut down on any coffee or tea that you drink and if possible, avoid emotional tension. If you know of special stress times that are unavoidable—such as Christmas, or exams, or even tax-paying time—you might want to visit your dermatologist for advice before the rosacea hits. Each flare-up weakens the vascular system and enlarges the blood vessels, leaving a permanent reminder of stress on your enlarged and reddened nose or face.

When washing your face, use only lukewarm or tepid water; avoid both extremes of hot and cold. Keep away from sun, bright lights, and sources of heat—hot ovens, radiators, and open fires. Think calm, blue-lavender thoughts, never flame-red ones.

Skin Stressors

Stress, especially the stress that is brought on by negative or self-demeaning thoughts, acts, or situations can affect the skin so adversely that it is doubtful that any skin-care program can overcome it. Like anything else, part of ridding yourself of skin problems is ridding yourself of the feeling that you don't look great! In fact, it is the first step. There is even an added plus to positive thinking: If you think you look terrific you will have more courage to try something new and daring. When you try something new, you gain self-confidence and that makes you look even better. It is a winning circle. The trick is to break into the circle and let it get rolling for you.

The following list of questions pinpoints some of the areas of self-esteem that you might want to think about and challenge. It is weighted toward your feelings about your own sexual attractiveness and your reactions to interpersonal relationships at work. These two areas seem to cause women more skin-stress than money management or other areas of adult adjustment. Write *yes* or *no* according to your own evaluation of yourself.

1. Do you spend more time thinking about the past than you spend planning for the future?
2. Are you afraid of disagreeing with your boss, or of bringing up a mistake you made, because you feel that you are being judged all the time?
3. Is it more than a month since you met someone new?
4. In the last few months have you fudged on your résumé, or led someone to believe that you had more influence, knowledge, or power than you actually have?
5. Do you secretly like to hear of someone in trouble, being fired, or being divorced?
6. Are you loath to show people how angry you really are, for fear of their retaliation?
7. Do you assign labels, such as "neurotic," to people who don't act in the way you think they should?
8. Do you make excuses to get out of going new places or doing new things that might put you in a vulnerable position?
9. Is it easier to reject people than admit that you might have mishandled the relationship?
10. Do you find that men are never as attentive or loving as you wish they would be?
11. Do you often find yourself relying on the prestige of your husband, lover, or family to impress new people?
12. Are there people in your neighborhood, office, or family that you don't speak to because of some disagreement?
13. Is it more than a month since you've given something to charity, or went out of your way to help someone?
14. Do you often go on diets, only to break them after a few days?
15. Do you ever feel alone and empty?

If you've answered yes to more than five of these questions, you're not as happy as you could be, and your skin probably isn't as happy as it could be. One of the ways of feeling better and more self-confident is getting control of yourself and your own life. One of the fastest, easiest ways of getting control is doing something that will reinforce your ability to change your own life for the better by changing another person's life —for the better. Right now: Do something small and simple that will make someone else happy. As soon as you can see their positive reaction it will tell you how powerful you are, and how much control you actually do have.

For example: Go out and buy someone you like a perfect apple. Yes, just an apple. (It is better than candy, because it cleans the teeth, sweetens the breath, and provides pectin for digestion.) Wrap the apple in crisp shiny foil, attach a bow, and give it with love. You'll see that this simple little "I like you" gift to anyone from the mail-person to a co-worker will make *you* sparkle, and will relieve your stress. It has to be a gift with no ulterior motives, and it has to be small and nonguilt evoking.

Many women are afraid that such small, gentle gestures will lead them down the road of the "passive patsy," but just the opposite is true. Just be sure that it is you who selects the gestures, and you'll find your skin condition, as well as your sleep, and your self-estimation will improve very fast.

Life in the Fast Lane Is Hard on Your Skin

The recent focus on career, health, and sports training may build muscle and self-esteem, but it has some harmful side-effects for many complexions. Adult acne is often caused by excess stress, compounded by mammoth mouthfuls of vitamins or health foods and some fast foods.

Megadoses of vitamins and pill-popping of mineral pills means that you are also taking in the large amounts of iodides and bromides that can cause pustular skin eruptions. Kelp, iodized salt, artichokes, spinach (yes, even the supposed wonder food), wheat germ, and shellfish all contain iodine. Wheat germ with a high yield of vitamin E can stimulate the sebaceous glands to secrete excessive amounts of oil. These glands can cause adult acne flare-ups.

Fast foods such as burgers and fries are also skin enemies. The food itself is not the problem, rather it is the harsh and excessive hygiene practiced in most fast-food restaurants that is the culprit. The equipment is cleaned with high-iodine solutions, some of which is then transferred to your food. If you have the choice, get broiled burgers rather than deep fried meats; the deep fryers seem to be cleaned most often with the highly saturated iodine solutions.

Besides staying away from megavitamins, unless they are prescribed by a doctor, some health foods, and some of your favorite seafoods, vegetables, and even diet pills, can cause complexion woes. They have been known to affect hormone levels and this can bring on acne. The diuretics in diet pills temporarily age the skin by making it flaky and crepy-looking.

Targeting Your Skin's Enemies

Here are four pictures. Each shows one of the stages of aging. Mark the stage that most closely represents your skin. Also mark any blemishes, discolorations, warts, or other skin problems that you have noticed. Show where the problem areas are located.

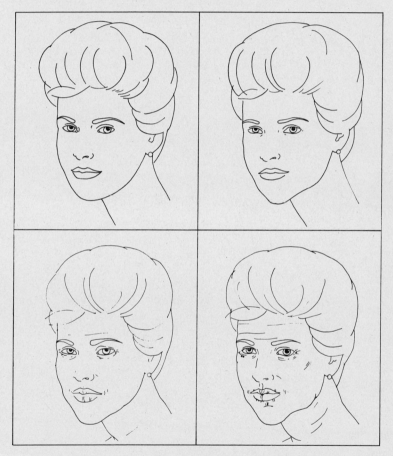

After you have marked the face-age chart you can make a daily plan for improving your skin. Don't be discouraged if you have indicated several skin problems—the skin can be regenerated, and you can start right now.

Harmful Products That Can Wreck Your Skin

To prevent damage to your complexion you should avoid:
— creams that contain hormones
— high alkaline creams
— perfume oils in lipstick
— lip glosses that are applied with the fingers
— metal lipstick containers that have nickel in them
— hair sprays that touch the ears
— bleaching and lightening creams with mercury

To prevent irritation and damage to your hair you should avoid:
— hair nets or caps with elastic bands
— detergents in shampoos
— nickel-plated curlers, hairpins, clips, or ornaments

To prevent irritation and damage to your hands you should avoid:
— soaps and detergents (wear rubber gloves whenever possible)
— ammonia in cleaners
— accumulations of soap under rings
— ribbons, carbon paper, NCR forms, scissors made of nickel
— acrylics
— formaldehyde in nail polish

To prevent damage or irritation to your eyes, or the eye area avoid:
— rubber sponges used to apply makeup
— eyeglass-cleaning solutions that contain silicone oils
— liquid mascara containing rosin
— eye shadow with powdered metals or fish scales
— eyebrow and eyelash dyes unless clearly approved by the FDA.

Sensitivity "Skindex"

Given enough abuse, even the strongest, thickest, youngest skin will wear and become irritated. People with sensitive skin have problems even if they constantly tend their skin with loving care. Usually sensitive skin is thinner and more delicate than the average, and probably has an allergic reaction to many substances. Most skin sensitivity is due to three factors: heredity, aging (older, thinner skin becomes increasingly sensitive to irritations that might not even cause a slight blush in our teens), and allergy.

Whether your skin is thick or thin, the number of oil glands and the activity of those glands are inherited characteristics. The people that seem most vulnerable to skin sensitivity are people of Celtic descent. They come from many regions in western Europe, and are often found in Ireland, Scotland, and northern Spain. Their thin, pale skin tends to burn rather than tan, and they are also vulnerable to broken capillaries because their skin is so thin that the tiny passages are easily affected by light and heat. Oriental women who have equally small oil glands do not usually have such sensitive skin because their skin is thicker and denser, and so stronger.

Black skin is very sensitive and it needs much gentler handling than white skin. Dark skin is very busy producing pigmentation and even a small scratch can leave a dark, irritated mark that will take months to heal. Black skin should be cleansed very carefully, and too-ambitious scrubbing with grains, a brush, or even a high-alcohol cleanser should be avoided because they keep black skin in a constant state of irritation that will make the skin uneven in color (the irritated sections tend to produce more color pigment).

No matter what sort of skin you have, you are suspectible to the drying effects of age and the environment. When skin is dry, and does not have sebum, it becomes tight and cracks, allowing irritants and allergy-producing chemicals to penetrate the skin's defenses. Be sure to cover your warm damp skin with a moisturizer right after you bathe, and before going out, especially as you get older. If you work near a radiator or other source of heat in the winter, you'll have to use moisturizer every few hours to keep your skin soft and supple and impermeable. Air conditioners pose the same risk.

Heredity is what you're born with; age is the effect of time on your genes; but allergies, although they may be triggered by heredity and age, are one of the most easily and successfully treated causes of sensitive skin. Rashes, itching areas, blotches, bumps, discolorations, and blemishes can all be part of allergic reactions. The reaction can weaken your skin, causing an infection that masks the allergic reaction. Be especially careful of new products such as sunscreens, perfumes, and ointments that contain lanolin, vitamin E, and benzocaine. These are substances that are known to cause allergic reactions in sensitive complexions.

Emotional stress, lack of sleep, and changes in routine, such as travel, seem to bring on allergic reactions. Perhaps it is because the body is less able to defend itself when under unusual strain. It is one of the reasons that allergies make your skin look its worst—just when you're under pressure to look or be your best. Exercise, gentle stimulation of the blood supply, and a positive outlook can do more to keep sensitive skin even and smoothly content than almost any other remedy.

You probably have been aware of adverse skin reactions from time to time, but you may not know whether your skin is unusually sensitive. This "Skindex" will help you rate your skin's sensitivity. Place a check in the column that best describes your skin's reactions:

	Always	Sometimes	Never
1. My eyes often feel itchy when I use a new cosmetic product.			
2. I have spells of sneezing, coughing, or even wheezing when I'm in an enclosed area.			
3. Some soaps make me red and make my skin taut.			
4. I've had strange rashes on my fingers and other parts of my body.			
5. My skin might suddenly go from smooth and creamy to red and sore.			
6. My lips often crack and peel when I try a new lipstick.			
7. I can't stand some fabrics because they make me feel itchy.			
8. There are often slight bumps under my skin, and I don't know why.			
9. On some days my skin gets chapped, sunburned, and peels after just a few minutes outside.			
10. I have a slight rash under the hook of my bra strap, and it never goes away.			

Give yourself 3 points for each Always answer, 2 for each Sometimes answer, and 1 for each Never answer. If you are fair, have thin skin, and sunburn easily, add 10 to your score. If you are over 30 years old, add another 10 to your score. If you've scored more than 25—you have sensitive skin!

Possible Allergens

If any cosmetic makes you feel itchy, or if your skin feels irritated or uncomfortable, or if it peels, becomes tender, or blotchy—you may be allergic to one of the ingredients in the cosmetic. Sometimes your skin won't react, but your eyes will feel tired and irritated.

Check the label of your cosmetic against this list of possible allergens. These ingredients have been known to be irritating to some people:

acacia
alizarin
alkaline earth sulfides
alum
aluminum sulphate
arrowroot
boric acid
cocoa butter
cornstarch
formaldehyde
gun arabic
gum tagacanth

hydroquinone
karaya gum
lanolin
lead
lycopodium
phenol
resorcinol
rice starch
salicylic acid
wheat starch
zinc chloride
zinc sulfate

OILS:
almond, bay, cottonseed,
coriander, eucalyptus,
lemon, linseed,
orange, wintergreen

This list certainly isn't complete; only you can know what ingredients might be harmful to you. Don't use anything that is suspect, however; you actually can make yourself more allergic by constant exposure.

How to Read a Label

All cosmetics that are sold in a state other than the one in which they were manufactured must list most of their ingredients. This list will tell you the chemical names for the substances in the order of their importance, or weight. You'll notice that many include "water" as the first listed ingredient; this is because water is the base of many skin-care products. If an ingredient is a drug, it is identified as an "active ingredient." Even a small amount of some active ingredients can make a big difference.

When manufacturers have a secret ingredient, they are not forced to reveal it; that ingredient can be listed under the heading "and other ingredients." Fragrances and flavors are also grouped together under general terms.

If an ingredient comprises less than 1 percent of the weight, it does not have to be listed in decreasing order, and there is no rule that forces a cosmetics manufacturer to indicate where the "less than 1 percent" ingredients begin on the label list.

Some private labels, stage makeup, and professional products require no label at all. In the case of mascara, the package is often so small that the ingredients must be listed on a little card or tag that is attached. Keep these tags; it is one cue to knowing if a reaction to a product might be caused by a specific ingredient.

If you suffer an adverse reaction to a cosmetic, you should report it to the manufacturer and send a copy of the letter to the Food and Drug Administration (also keep a copy for yourself). When you write, describe the product and identify it by any letters or numbers so it can be traced by the batch. Be sure to describe the problem or symptoms, say how long they lasted, and if medical treatment was necessary include proof of the treatment, such as a copy of any prescription. Address the letter to the Food and Drug Administration, Division of Cosmetic Technology, 5600 Fishers Lane, Rockville, MD 20857.

Simple Patch Tests for Cosmetics

If that wonderful new makeup base that looked so fabulous when you put it on looks less fabulous after a few days, or if your skin suddenly starts to feel tender and uncomfortable, or if your eyes tear, your nose tickles, and you start sneezing: check your cosmetics for possible allergic reaction.

You should really test every cosmetic before you use it, but in reality, most people are just so anxious to see how wonderful they'll look that they rush right home to try the product. Very few have patience enough to wait the necessary two days for an at home sensitivity test, although it's very easy to do, and could save your skin damaging irritation. Here is the simplest way of testing your cosmetics to be sure they are not irritating to your skin:

— Decide where the test will be. The best sites are the upper arm and neck.
— Clean the skin of the test site very carefully; dry it well.
— Take a bit of the cream or makeup and put it on a small piece of gauze, or saturate a small piece of cotton with it.
— Tape it to the inside of your upper arm, near your armpit, or tape it to the side of your neck, if your hair will cover the test.
— Leave the patch of the cosmetic you are testing untouched for at least 48 hours.
— Remove the tape and gauze carefully and examine the skin.

If your skin is red, blotchy, or irritated where the cosmetic touched it, the cosmetic is probably not for you. Discard the makeup or cosmetic no matter how much you paid for it—it will do your skin (and your looks) more harm than good.

Sportscare for Skin

Dehydration can be almost as damaging to the skin as are the effects of the sun. During the summer's heat or in a heated gym, you lose both salt and water as you perspire, especially if you are exercising.

You can take some precautions that will help get the best skin-improving results from your activities. After exposure to the sun, use Cetaphil Lotion, which is relatively inexpensive and acts as a skin cleanser. It can be bought at most pharmacies. You can also soothe sun-baked skin with cold compresses made of milk or with cooled tea leaves or tea bags. These are standard folklore remedies—and they do provide relief.

Swimmers are especially vulnerable to the effects of the sun because they often forget to reapply sun-block cream, and because they forget that the sun's rays can reach them through the water.

Pool swimmers offend their skin with chlorine and other highly alkaline disinfectants, and lake and surf swimmers—especially off some of our tropical shores—do not protect themselves against stings and rashes of sea creatures and plants as well as rough sandy shores. If you do encounter a jellyfish, or notice an itchy rash after swimming, use light alcohol on the area. You can use witch hazel, cologne, or even vodka, but don't use plain water.

Dr. James Baral, a New York dermatologist, is an avid athlete who walks about 15 miles a day. He stresses the importance of proper sports clothing for comfort and skin protection. "Tennis players, joggers, and aerobic exercisers or dancers should always wear clothing that will absorb perspiration, and cotton socks that will keep the feet dry," advises Baral. "Use thong sandals in public locker rooms, or around pools to protect against such funguses as athlete's foot, and use common sense and moderation when you're staying fit."

Women are especially vulnerable to skin damage and to damaging or weakening the connective tissue and skin collagen when they are exercising, jogging, or jumping rope. Each step or jump brings the force of gravity into play. The large, heavy, or weak areas of the body and face, such as the buttocks, the breasts, and the chin, that are not supported are literally hurled downward with almost every downward motion of the body. Sagging breasts, sinking fannies, and loose chins result.

The firm sports bra is the best way to ensure no damage to connective tissue on the sides of the breasts. Entertainers and dancers have always had their costumes carefully fitted, just to protect their bodies. Elastic pants, not too different from the old-fashioned girdle, can help if you have a very large bottom. The chin should also be protected. A chin strap of a soft material, even a cotton or linen hanky held tight by an elastic ribbon, works very well. Wide elastic ribbons, the kind used by seamstresses for skirt-waists covered with a pleasant-looking soft decorative ribbon, will look very much like a misplaced headband and be a valuable face-saver if you jog or jump rope.

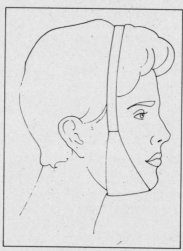

Chin Strap

5

Create the Face
You Want

Makeup may not be one of the basic necessities of life, like food or shelter, but it can change the quality of your life. Others respond to the you they see, and you also think of yourself in visual terms. Recent improvements in the formulations of makeup have also turned cosmetics into protective creams, such as makeup foundations with built-in sunscreen. In a study published in 1984, Jean Ann Graham and Albert M. Kligman of the University of Pennsylvania's School of Dermatology reported experimental evidence showing that the use of cosmetics improves the way we feel about ourselves and the way others feel about us. Groups of participants were given cosmetic make-overs and changes were measured in their appearance, socializing, feelings, self-images, outlook, and attitudes. Short- and long-term self-perception improved. The researchers noted that the women who wore cosmetics were perceived by others to have better personalities than women who did not use them.

There is usually very little difference between the formulas for inexpensive and expensive creams and moisturizers. This is also usually true for makeup. Although the higher-priced cosmetics' makers are able to bring out new shades that are better suited to current fashions, and the colors are more appealing and richer-looking in the cases or jars, it is possible to find dime-store brands that are as good or better—for you and the look you want—than the most expensive makeups. More important than brand, or even color, seems to be the ability to use makeup. It is like the story of Pablo Picasso who was able in just moments, with a few crayons or ordinary pencils, to create a work of timeless art. It wasn't his tools or palette—it was how he used them.

Foundations

The right foundation for you will protect your skin, even the tone and color, and act as a base (a foundation) for other makeup.

Most foundations contain anywhere from 40 to 75 percent water, depending on the form of the foundation. The balance of ingredients is color (white to deep umber), oils to soothe the skin and provide a vehicle for the color, and some "barrier" chemicals such as zinc oxide. Most foundations also include a humectant—a substance that attracts moisture from the air—such as glycerine or urea. This keeps the foundation fresh-looking because it keeps it moist, and it also keeps the skin under the foundation moist.

Don't hesitate to apply two different brands, or types, of foundation to your skin. If you have dry spots or oily areas, switch foundations and treat each section of your face separately. It takes a few minutes to blend the foundations together so they meet invisibly; but your makeup will look better—and last longer.

Foundations are available in a large variety of textures and hundreds of colors. A complete "foundation wardrobe" should include four or five different products—all in the smallest size possible. Included should be a basic shade as well as one shade lighter and one shade darker in an oil-base foundation, and a foundation in your basic color in a water base.

To find the right basic shade, select a color that blends well with the skin along your jawline, just under your ear. Once you've found the right color there will be no difference between the makeup itself and the color of your skin on your jaw and neck. Most people are urged to buy foundation that is too dark or too rosy for them. A darker color will not give more coverage; it will just make you look slightly dirty.

To apply the foundation, dot cream or liquid base over the face, starting in the middle of the face. Spot the foundation on nose, chin, upper lip, and forehead first, then inner cheeks, and finally—without adding more foundation to your fingers—stroke the dots outward. In that way the foundation will be concentrated where it is most needed, and taper off so that it will not cake at the hairline or get on your hair. Most professional artists use a small latex or natural sponge, dampened with water, but most women find fingertips easier.

Different types of foundation serve different purposes:

Liquid Base	is the most popular because it is easy to apply. The color is usually suspended in an oil base, provides medium coverage, and needs a dusting of powder for a matte finish.
Water base	foundation must be shaken thoroughly to blend the color and oils with the water. It is difficult to apply evenly because it is so watery. There is usually an antibacterial or other antiseptic in the emulsion. Even if you have oily skin use this sparingly; this medicated water base may be too harsh for your eye area and your throat.
Whipped bases	are light in texture but offer little coverage. They're light, oily, and go on easily, but leave little but a shine. Wonderful for the woman with a perfect complexion who doesn't need any makeup.
Translucent gels	are very popular with men who just want to even skin color; these give very little coverage.
Matte bases	have a tendency to clog pores, and also to cake on dry skin. In theory they give a velvety smoothness, but they are really just a cream base, with additional powder, packaged in a tube. Even the smoothest skin will look withered if this base is applied too heavily.
Pressed powder cake	offers heavy coverage and a cakey texture. Touch-ups just encourage caking. These are usually sold as a convenient way of keeping your makeup fresh all day. Adding the powder dries the makeup and absorbs skin oils. Instead, just spray makeup with water.
Cream stick	gives a smooth heavy coverage; it provides a lasting, all-day foundation. Because it is so thick, it is best applied to a wet face that is primed with a light coat of moisturizer.
Cake base	is water soluble and is applied with a damp sponge. It is excellent for oily skin because it is a water-base product. It can be freshened easily with a damp sponge, rather than applying additional makeup.

Foundation for a Sculpted Look

Foundations can do more than just provide even coverage; using a variety of shades of foundation to create an illusion of depth or to highlight isn't new. Foundations are ideal contour-makers, and are good concealers, too. *Max Factor's Pan Stik Makeup* is a great nose-maker because it absorbs the excess oil on the nose, and is in a form that is easy to apply in a controlled manner. Foundations are also less pore-clogging than concealers, or even sculpture sticks.

Nose To detract attention from a large nose, apply a darker foundation on the sides of the nose; use a light foundation on the cheeks. Keep the blusher on the outer edges of the face. For a wide nose, streak a lighter foundation down the top, stopping before you reach the tip. Narrow wide nostrils by applying a darker foundation to both sides of the nostrils.

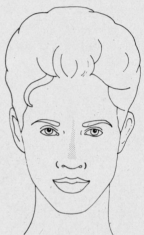

Wide Nose and Wide Nostrils

Forehead   Raise a low forehead by blending a succession of light foundations upward from the brows. Keep the lightest section near the hairline. Broaden a narrow forehead by lightening the temple area. A bulging or uneven forehead can be minimized by using a slightly darker foundation on the enlarged area.

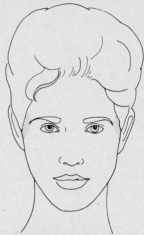

Narrow Forehead

Jaw   To tone down a broad jaw, apply a darker shade over the widest area. If your jawline is narrow, you can strengthen it by using a lighter foundation at the edge of the jaw.

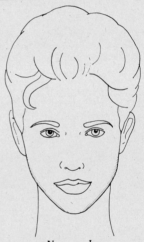

Narrow Jaw

Neck

To slim a thick neck, use a foundation that is slightly darker than the one you use on your face. If your neck is too thin, lighten the edges with a skin bleach, and use a light-toned foundation.

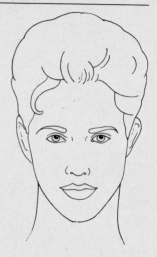

Thick Neck

Chin

To balance a long, strong chin that dominates the face, shadow the chin with a darker foundation. To enlarge a small chin, coat with a light foundation. Minimize a sagging or double chin with a darker foundation.

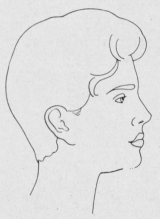

Double Chin

Ears   Narrow a broad face by shading the sides and the ears in a darker foundation. Broaden a narrow face with a light foundation, and lighten ears and lobes.

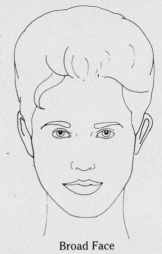

Broad Face

Powders

The problem with powder is that it changes color on the face because the powder hasn't been matched with the acid/alkaline balance of the skin. If your brush or puff turns orange after a few days' use, you can be sure that the powder is also turning orangish after several hours on your face. Loose powder is a perennial favorite because there is nothing that makes the skin look as velvety, smooth, and poreless as powder. A light, natural look in powder is favored by most women. ,

Powders are available in loose, or pressed, form. The pressed powders are really thickened foundations, and they cake easily. Loose powders should be puffed or brushed on with a brush, feather, or cottony puff as evenly as possible. Transparent powder is used to give your makeup a matte finish with no change or added color from the powder itself. The basic ingredients are kaolin, a kind of clay, and zinc stearate, to maximize coverage. Thick powders can be drying; they act just as kaolin does in a face mask, they absorb the facial oil. Powder can actually draw the moisture from your skin.

When powdering your face, start at the chin and outer edges (the opposite way than you do foundation). The reason is that if your nose is oily, all the powder will just cake up on the oily nose. Applying powder to a shiny nose will just create mud—rather, apply cool water, blotted on with a sponge. The shine will vanish.

Is Your Powder Doing Its Job?

How can you tell which powder is best for you? What does a "good" powder look like? How will it go on? The powder that is right for your skin will—

- Have a smooth feel to the skin, it will "slip" on easily and be composed of very fine particles.
- Adhere to your skin—with or without a creamy foundation to hold it; once brushed on, it will stay on.
- Absorb oils, perspiration, or other moisture on your skin. Some powders are too absorbent and dry the skin; others are washed away by skin oils.
- Cover shine, enlarged pores, discolorations, and defects.
- Seem to give a plush or velvet surface to the skin, so the skin doesn't seem plastic or too slick.
- Provide an even, unchanging color to the skin that will remain on the surface of the skin, blending with the foundation.
- Have a fragrant odor, but not be too perfumed.

Concealers

These products are more opaque and should be lighter in color than your foundation. They are used in an effort to counteract any dark areas of the skin—dark circles, shadows, blemishes, and dramatically uneven pigmentation. The problem with concealers is that they are difficult to apply properly and require a very light touch to blend them. Although professional makeovers in magazines and in stores show exactly how to do this, it is an art that is difficult to duplicate when you are rushing to get dressed and get to work on time.

Most concealers are available in small thick sticks, or as skin-colored lipsticks. In either case, they are difficult to apply to a thin wrinkle, or line, and stick to your fingers when you try to smudge them and blend them. This is an example of a cosmetic being only as good as your technical ability to handle it. The following technique works well with almost everyone:

Apply the concealer with a thin sable paintbrush. Stroke it directly on the crease or over the area to be obscured. Tap the skin gently to even out and blend the color, then dot on a slightly lighter color of the same foundation that you will apply to your face. Apply your foundation, and carefully blend the two colorations together without wiping off the concealer. Many makeup artists prefer to apply concealer over foundation; they feel less concealer is used, and there are fewer clogged pores.

Concealers are often used in combination with contours and blushers. Lightening one area of the face and darkening another creates a much more subtle effect than using only a contour.

Side Views

Most people apply makeup looking directly into a well-lighted mirror. This gives them a full-face view of themselves, but that isn't the view that most of your audience will see. Most people are seen more often in profile than in full-face, and although it is more difficult to see yourself that way, it is well worth the angled mirrors and the neck twisting. You'd look pretty silly with only the front of your hair combed, or with the back of your skirt hem dragging—the same goes for your makeup.

The ideal profile is perpendicular. To test your side view use a wooden ruler and place it against your face resting on your brow bone, covering one eye, and then slanting slightly to rest on your chin. Does it tilt, or does it remain perpendicular to the floor? If it tilts outward at the chin, your chin is too prominent. (Marilyn Monroe had her chin made more prominent through plastic surgery. It changed her career.) You can use contour and blusher to sculpt your face so that it appears in proportion.

Dominant Chin Soften the chin, jawline, and the forehead by using a slightly darker-than-natural foundation. Tip the nose with a light concealer and blend the highlighter up the bridge of the nose.

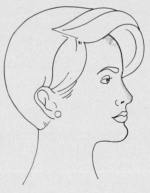

Weak Chin   Cover the edge of the chin with a highlighter to bring it forward and blend well up the jawline.

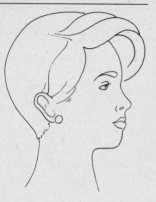

Weak Forehead   If your head slopes backward, you can correct the illusion by covering the upper part of the forehead with a highlighter. If your forehead is narrow, use a horizontal band near the hairline; if your forehead is wide, keep highlighter centered.

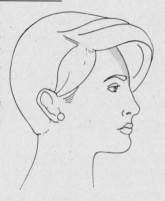

The shape of your skull has just as many variations as your other facial features. The oval or egg shape is considered ideal for the face; from chin to the top of your crown, your profile should be even and graceful. Most problems in head shape can be disguised easily with a variation in hairstyle.

Blush/Contours

The image of health and vitality has replaced the look of the youthful embarrassed blush, or the pallid femme fatale, and so blusher has replaced rouge and contours have replaced a flat, chalky complexion.

Blushers are made of the same ingredients as pressed face powders and eye shadows, except the color range goes from warm browns through reds into mauves and pinks, with none of the blues and greens of eye shadow. The major ingredients are still water (although there is less of it than in a foundation), oils, waxes, gels, and colorants.

Blushers are mixed blessings because they impart a look of health, but often make the wearer look older because the color deepens in the small cracks of rough or wrinkled skin, accentuating the flaws. Cream rouge or cream blusher can also make small pit scars from ancient acne problems more noticeable because the color fills the tiny holes. The ideal blusher will cover tiny imperfections with a velvety finish and blend perfectly with the natural color of the skin, so the color seems to come from within the skin rather than over the surface.

Cream blusher does last longer than the dry version, and retains its original color longer, but it is more difficult to apply evenly and correctly and to feather out and blend. Gels and color contour pencils are a recent innovation in the old problem of getting the color where you want, and making it stay there, but neither work as well as the powdery blusher and brush technique. Pencils (sometimes called crayons because of their size) are waxy and difficult to apply without pulling and smearing on the skin. The gels cause a problem because they dry so quickly, and because they are water-based they have a drying effect on the skin. Gels also fill in large pores, pitted scars, and wrinkles very fast, and seem to work well only on fair, youthful skin.

Contours are actually blushers, they are just somewhat deeper and more shadowy in color than blushers. The theory of contours is that light colors advance, and deep or dark colors look like hollows. The camera can often be fooled by the use of contours to "model" a face, but the human eye cannot. Applying contours and blushers is much harder than it looks, because although anyone can do it, few are really sure they're doing it right.

Is Your Blusher Right for You?

Is it easy to control and apply?

Does the color last for several hours?

Does the color blend easily without looking obvious?

Is it smooth and even-textured?

Does it disappear after a few hours?

Is the color harsh?

Are you never sure you have used enough,
   until you have too much on?

Does it leave a greasy or unnatural glow?

If you answered *yes* to the first four questions, and *no* to the second four, you and your blusher are perfectly matched. If not, it may not be your blusher's fault. Blusher should be the focus of the eye, and should counteract any out-of-proportion facial feature, as well as giving a healthy glow. Here is how to apply a blusher to get its best effects:

Oval face   Apply in a triangular shape with the apex of the triangle pointing to mid-nose; starting under the pupil, blend well toward the temple and jaw.

Long or Narrow Face   Apply in a short rectangular shape, going from earlobe to mid-cheek. Don't get too near the nose; the effect will be a pinched and narrow look. Think horizontal.

Heavy Jaw   Use a light contour or concealer on the temples to make the forehead appear broader, and use blush or contour as a vertical stripe from the outer corner of the eye, down the face to the edge of the jaw. Blend the dark concealer or blusher along the jawline slightly. Think narrow.

Square Jaw   Take the corners off the square by using blush on the upper temples, blended into the hairline, and on the jaw from mid-ear to bottom of the jaw.

Narrow Jaw   Blend upward and on the sides of the eyes and
                          temple. Keep the blusher very high on the face.
                          Use a line of lighter than natural color base along
                          the jawline to make it appear stronger and firmer.

Round Face   Apply blusher to the outer edges of the face. Tip
                          the chin with a light foundation to make it appear
                          stronger and draw attention away from the wide
                          cheeks.

Diamond Face   Starting at the outer edges of the eye, and moving
                          toward the temple and ear, stroke the blusher out-
                          ward. Use highlighter on the temples and on the
                          jaw.

As Dr. Diana Bihova, a dermatologist with extensive knowledge of cosmetics, points out, powdered blusher is more suitable for very hot
weather than cream blushers or rouges; the oils in the creams become
less stable when they are exposed to heat. She suggests using lip pencils
and powder blushers on the beach. The colorants also act as a sun de-
flector.

Shadows and Glitters

Makeup for the eyes. A shadow can create the illusion of a violet or green iris, can make your eyes look larger, rounder, almond shaped, and more lustrous than you imagined possible. But eye makeup is also the most difficult cosmetic to apply correctly, because the area is so crowded naturally, and because the color must be selected to fit your hair, eyes, complexion, and clothing.

Choose a color that complements your clothing and *contrasts* with the color of your eyes. If you're wearing blue, and have blue eyes, then select a green or violet, something that will play up the blue of your eyes. If you have brown eyes, use blue- or gray-toned shadows.

Shadows and glitters should never look patchy or uneven. The effect you want is smooth, pearly color. To achieve this, blend shadows with an up-and-down movement, using a soft watercolor brush, a tiny sponge, or a cotton swab. Don't pull or drag the skin. By its very nature, shadow is difficult to remove, and the act of removing it is very stressful for your skin. George Masters, a Hollywood makeup maven, believes that each time you remove eye shadow you subject this thin skin to a trauma that causes early sags and bags.

To keep shadows adhering to the eyelid, use a bit of foundation on the lid to "fit" the powder or cream color, and dust around the eye with loose powder. The color is a matter of personal taste, and of fashion, but there are some general guidelines: smoky colors for day, glitter for evening. If you want to use more than one color, use the lightest shade on the inner half of the lid, nearest the eye; the darker or darkest shade on the crease, under the brow bone, and extend it outward to the outer part of the lid. Blend all the colors carefully.

Eye Openers

You can sculpt your face by highlighting your eyes with a dot of white or very light beige on the eyelids up toward the brow. Place the dot on the inner corner of the eye for a round face, and near the outer corner for a narrow face.

Applying the shadow properly can change the illusion of the size and shape of the eye.

Small Eyes	Light color on the lids and outward. Darker color above, in the crease, extended outward. If the face is wide at the temples, do not extend the light from the lids very far beyond the outer edge.
Close-set Eyes	If there is less than an "eye's length" between your eyes, your eyes are too close-set. A high bridge nose can also make your eyes look close-set. Cover the entire inner eye area and nose with a light shadow, or a concealer.
Wide-set Eyes	If your eyes are small and your nose bridge is flat, you can create an illusion of depth by shading the inner corners of the eye and using a dark contour on the sides of the bridge of the nose. Keep the outer edges of the eyes light.
Sad Eyes	Extend the darkest shadow across the upper lid and create a light area just under the brow. The creation of a horizontal dark area will make the eyes look less tilted.
Bulging Eyes	A heavy brow helps to balance protruding eyes. Shade the midsection of the eyelid with a dark color, and blend that shadow upward. The entire eye area should be lightly shaded to make the orbs recede.
Narrow or Oriental Eyes	To create a feeling of depth and drama use a highlight under the eyes, and also on the entire brow bone. Create depth in the eye by darkening the area just above the crease, and dotting a bit of highlight on the center of the upper and lower lids.

Another tip about shadow removal: Carefully dot a light vegetable oil around the eye, over the shadow. Blot the oil and color off together by applying a folded tissue to the shadowed area. Keep oiling and blotting; try not to move the skin or even the eyelid. Wiping will not hurt once or twice—but moving the skin every day has a cumulative effect.

Eyeliners and Rims

Applying eye makeup is influenced by two things: the shape of your eyes, and the amount of space around your eyes, between your two eyes, between your brow and lashes, and between your eye and cheekbone.

Eyeliners are used to accentuate or change the actual shape of your eyes. They are usually available in pencils, liquid, cake form (applied with a very thin, tiny sable brush), or a newer pencil brush. Eyeliner can be used with shadow, with mascara, with both, or alone. Waterproof liner must be removed with oil or a cream.

The eyeliner should be applied at the roots of the lashes, or as near as possible to the very base of the lashes. Don't extend the line beyond the inner corner of the eye, and never extend it in thick wings over the outer eyelid. Correctly applied, eyeliner can make ordinary eyes look fabulous.

Liner is a bit tricky, and there are ways of making a neat, mistake-proof line more easily. Place a small mirror or a hand mirror flat on a table or a level surface that is even with the bottom of your nose. Look downward, through your lashes; you should be able to see your upper lip and the base of your lashes in the mirror.

Start at the outer corner and work inward. Do not, as most directions tell you, hold or pull your lid taut. Just draw a line inward toward the inner end of the top lid. If your eyes are

close-set, stop slightly before the center of the eye
almond-shaped, make the bottom line darker than the top
wide-set, line the full top lid and the outer half of the lower lid
bloodshot or tired, try a white or blue line on the inner edge of the
   lower lid

One of the newest techniques in applying eyeliner is to dot the liner rather than draw it in a smooth unbroken line. Smudge each dot slightly. To smudge the liner, use a flat toothpick with one end wrapped in a tiny bit of cotton or a cotton swab. (Obviously a new one is needed for each application to avoid bacteria growth.) This technique works well for pencil eyeliner, but does not work for liquid liner; attempting to smudge a liquid will make it flake off.

Applying eye liner pencil on the little ledge inside the lashes is popular with the steady-handed, but it often leads to conjunctivitis.

Mascara

Many women consider mascara their most important cosmetic. It can do more for the morale, and for an ultra-luxurious look, than any other cosmetic. Mascara is available in many forms:

Cake comes in small rectangles with small brushes for application. Many people think this is best; you can moisten the cake and get exactly the consistency you want. But you should *never* wet the cake with saliva, and you should wash the brush carefully after each use (although no one I've ever met—me included—ever does).

Creme mascara is sold in small tubes. It is nice and thick, and many women find it gives good coverage, although it has a tendency to gob on lash tips.

Liquid is sold in small bottles with tiny comb applicators; several coats are often needed.

Roll-on, in a thick liquid, with a spiral or straight brush applicator that fits in the dispenser, is the most popular. Lash-builder mascaras contain tiny filaments almost like the plush of velvet, which are cut free and suspended in the colored liquid. These tiny fibers stick to the lashes when the mascara dries and make the lashes longer and thicker.

Waterproof mascara must be removed with oil.

Eyelash dyes and eyebrow dyes are made of highly purified chemical dyes. They come in limited colors. They must be used only by professionals, and many people hesitate to use them because they fear allergic reactions.

Apply mascara to all of your lashes, upper and lower.

1. Lower your top lids about halfway. Apply mascara to the top side of the upper lid's lashes.
2. Then slightly tilt head back and open eyes wide. Apply mascara to the underside of the upper lashes.
3. Use an even stroke and bring the brush from the base to the tips.
4. Then, with the brush newly loaded, double and triple coat the tips of the lashes, spreading the mascara with a horizontal move from the tips of the lashes around the inner eye to the tips of the lashes at the outer eye. Repeat from the outer tips to the inner, several times.
5. Allow lash tips to dry slightly.
6. Powder lashes very lightly and repeat mascara application.

7. Allow top lashes to dry completely.
8. Tilt the head forward slightly; look downward.

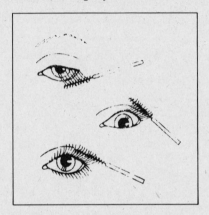

9. Coat only outer sides of the bottom lashes in the same way as the top, first from base to tip, then tips only in a horizontal movement.
10. Finally coat both the upper and lower lashes one last time.

If your lashes stick together or the mascara beads on the lashes, use a flat wooden toothpick to separate the lashes. Gently, using a slight sawing motion, cut through the caked lashes. And do it immediately, before the mascara dries. If the mascara does dry, sticking the lashes together, wrap the end of the toothpick in cotton, wet the cotton (oil for waterproof mascara), and very gently melt the dry mascara and separate the lashes.

If your lower lashes curl onto your lower lids and dot them with the wet mascara, simply use a slip of paper under your lashes as you apply the mascara. Clean any mascara spots or mistakes immediately. The longer you wait, the more difficult cleanup becomes; and when mascara dries, it becomes almost impossible. However, a cotton-wrapped toothpick, used with a twirling motion, helps.

Lipstick/Lip Color

Lip color is the most popular of all makeup. It has made a strong come-back after being ignored a dozen or so years ago. Even men have been using lip glosses and balms or ointments to keep their lips kissable.

Most lip colors are a mixture of wax (for the base of the stick), oil (usually castor oil), and some color pigments. The pigment is the vital ingredient because lipstick is blatant color. For years blue-reds were out and wines and red-browns were favored. Recently, pinks and fuschia have become popular. The color should be bright and pure without being harsh.

The complaint that most women have is that lipstick seems to vanish in an hour or two. The "better" looking the lipstick, the faster it will disappear. If you wear a long-lasting lipstick you'll find that it often changes color on the lips. This is due to the mixing of various pigments; some last longer than others.

Lips are different from skin in other parts of the body. They are mucous membrane and have no upper layer to act as a protective barrier, neither do they have the ability to create melanin, the body's natural skin coloring. Because of this they are very vulnerable. And, lips that are dry, chapped, and peeling defy cosmetic coverage.

If your lips tend to dry, cover them with a specially formulated product such as Blistex. This will prevent evaporation of the skin's natural moisture, and will avoid additional evaporation because it will stop you from licking your own lips. One of the problems with lip health is the dry lips make you want to moisten them, so you lick them, coating them with saliva. This quickly evaporates and dries the skin even more—setting up a wet/dry cycle which can irritate your lips. Luckily restoring injured lips to good health is relatively easy because a strong blood supply makes them heal very quickly.

Corrective Lip Makeups

It's fairly easy to correct your lip shape to be very close to your ideal. What isn't easy is getting the lip color to stay where you want it—crisp, clean-edged, and fresh. You can extend the life of your lip color from minutes to hours, even after eating and drinking, simply by using a moisturizer and makeup foundation on your lips under the lipstick or lip color.

After a "primer" coat of foundation you're ready for the color. Use a pencil or a lip brush to outline your lips. You should actually draw the outline of the shape you want. A pencil works best for full or older lips, a brush for thinner or younger lips. The pencil leaves a waxy barrier that holds the color in place. Be bold—experiment. Don't worry about being extreme. Changing your lip line is one of the most correctable of all cosmetic changes; if you don't like it, simply wash it away.

Thin upper lip   Create a new lip line slightly above your natural one, but be very aware of the length of the area between nose and mouth. If you have a short upper lip, or a very long chin, it is best to leave the upper lip the way it is.

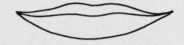

Thin lower lip   Extend the color below the lip line. If your jaw is narrow, keep the lower lip fairly straight and horizontal. If your jaw is wide, keep the fullness directly over the chin in the center of your lips. Don't extend the curve of lower lip downward if your chin is small or weak—it will make the chin seem to vanish altogether.

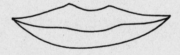

Both lips are thin   Increase the size of both lips, but if your mouth is narrow, extend the lip line slightly at the edges to avoid a pouty look.

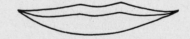

Downward corners   As the skin sags around the mouth, the corners of your mouth seem to droop, making you look tired, angry, and old. Lift the corners by drawing an upward tilt at each corner of the upper lip.

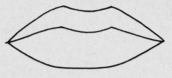

Small mouth   Extend the outer corners. For a large mouth, stop the lines before reaching the outer corner.

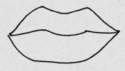

Uneven lips   Very few people have symmetrical, perfect lips. Fill in areas that are too small with color, and go lightly on over-full areas. Distract attention from your mouth to one of your more perfect features. For example, play up nice ears with an off-the-face hairstyle and fantastic earrings.

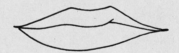

Oval mouth   If your "Cupid's bow" isn't well-defined and curved, you can create one by drawing a "V" from two points on the furrow on your upper lip to the bottom middle of your upper lip. Fill in the "V" with color until you have the effect you want.

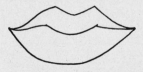

After outlining your lips with a brush or pencil, fill in the color with a lipstick or the brush. Blotting your lips lightly on a tissue and then applying a second coat is a good way to extend the life of lip color. A matte finish will last longer than a glossy finish.

While you're working on correcting the size or shape of your lips, be aware of their position on your face. The most picture-perfect painted lips will not look right unless they are part of the balance and symmetry of your other features. A bold mouth must be balanced by strong eyes and brows—or you'll look fishy. And always keep in mind the shape of your jaw as you redraw and adapt your lips.

Lip-Smooth

Some of the most irritating and aging wrinkles are really tiny ones. They are very noticeable because these tiny vertical lines appear around the mouth. Lipstick "bleeds" into these cracks, calling attention to them. With a program of care and exercise these lines can be softened or erased, and feathered lip lines and dry cracked lips can be a thing of the past.

These small lines can develop because the skin between the upper lip and the nose is very thin. It is often supported by active hair follicles, but when that hair is bleached, waxed, or removed in any way, the skin weakens. Women who have had electrolysis on their upper lips often report a tendency to wrinkle after the hair is removed. There is also a tendency to forget about the upper lip when applying moisturizer or creams.

Here are several methods of fighting these lines. They all work—a little. Together, they can make a real difference in your lip line in just a few weeks:

Smoothing the Lines:

1. Coat the upper lip and mouth with cod-liver oil, or a thick vegetable oil, such as avocado oil.
2. Dip the little finger of one hand in granulated sugar. (Use the little finger because it is the weakest.)
3. Very gently rub the sugar across the lines on the upper lip. Then circle the mouth.
4. Wash away the sugar with warm water. Allow the oil to remain several hours or overnight.

Recently special products for the lips have become very popular. They work very well because they seal in lips and allow the skin to heal itself. At the same time they form a sort of primer-coat under the lipstick that makes smooth, even application of lipstick and a non-feathering lip-line possible. You can use any one of these products, and you can also avoid the problem by using moisturizer on the skin of your upper lip, and on the area around your mouth.

Pressing the Lines Flat:

1. Coat the upper lip and mouth with cod-liver oil, or a thick vegetable oil.
2. Apply a small piece of plastic wrap over the mouth. It will stick to the oil.
3. Using your index or middle finger, pat the plastic gently to urge the oil into the skin.
4. Pat gently for about a minute.
5. Relax and allow the oil to sink in for about 5 minutes more.
6. Strip off the plastic; rinse the face with warm water. The skin above your lip will seem plumper, and the wrinkles will have receded.

Stamp Out Wrinkles

Pasting stamps on the upper lip will temporarily erase the small wrinkles on the upper lip.

Lip-Smooth Cream

Mix together in a small jar or empty lip-gloss container a teaspoon of petroleum jelly, a teaspoon of coconut oil, and half of a small lipstick-size commercial lip-balm. Use this night and morning, coating your upper lip and the area between nose and lip.

Lip-Proof

To prevent lipstick from bleeding outline your lips with a dry lip pencil. Fill in the lip area with a creamier lipstick or a colored lip gloss.

Dr. Charles Zugerman, of Northwestern University Medical School, and a consultant to Blistex, suggests using a lip-balm that contains a sunscreen. He says, "Sunlight can have a profound effect on the collagen which gives the skin body and resilience, and actually holds it together. Just as collagen gradually changes with aging both men and women, so too a similar process occurs when the sun beats down on unprotected lips—accounting for wrinkled lips and fine lines around the mouth." (Blistex provides lip-tips in an informational booklet that is free if you write to Blistex Inc. Oak Brook, Illinois, 60521.)

Cold Sores (Herpes Simplex)

This viral infection can cause recurrent blisters on your lips or the edges of your lips. It affects a large percentage of the population, and only dental cavities and the common colds seem to be more of a problem.

Once the virus is contracted it can exist in a latent state through your life, or show itself during times of stress, such as when you have a cold, or just days before a menstrual period, or if you're very tired; sometimes it just occurs at regular intervals. It will frequently appear on the upper tip of the upper lip, or on the outer edges of the lower lip. An allergic reaction, such as a reaction to toothpaste, can trigger a herpes eruption.

Besides being unpleasant in appearance, the breakage in the skin caused by herpes can invite a bacterial infection and add to the problem.

There are numbers of medications and methods of treatment, and scientists are looking for a complete cure. Medications that include camphor make the tender area less sensitive and promote drying of the blister crust, and those that include menthol and zinc oxide promote healing and prevent further infection. The best thing you can do is to avoid an outbreak, and that means avoiding excessive exposure to sun, wind, and glare, and avoiding any irritation to the lip area, and mouth.

Warning: the herpes virus seems to be very determined, and there is evidence that it can live for a short time on a lipstick. Avoid using "tester" lipsticks in department and drugstores.

Teeth

Smooth skin, glossy lashes, and sparkling eyes add up to good looks, but you need pearly teeth to complete the picture. As we age, our teeth change, too. Although adults are less prone to cavities, they are more prone to gum problems. As the skin ages, so too do the gums. They become less firm, less elastic, and they shrink. They start to recede, which exposes more of the teeth. The expression "long of tooth" to describe someone of advanced age is very appropriate.

Years of careless tooth care can come home to roost, much in the same way oversunning takes its toll years later; and V-shaped grooves start to appear on the gum line. The shrunken and receding gums do not support the lips as well as they once did, and so the upper lip, which is also thinning, is too big for the mouth, and small lines appear running from the edge of the upper lip toward the nose. The use of oils or creams on the upper lip help, but preserving the teeth and firming the gums are the best ways to prevent these wrinkles.

When your teeth, gums, and mouth are not properly cleaned after eating, small bits of food remain between the teeth. The material decays and breeds masses of bacteria, commonly called *plaque*. Sensitive, bleeding gums are a sign of trouble. No technique, lip brush, color, or special gloss can make up for a decayed tooth. And certainly the foul breath that is part of the infection is an enemy of beauty.

Plaque is difficult to see because it takes on the coloration of the healthy tissue, but it can easily be seen if the teeth are stained with special dyes. There are some commercial dyes you can find at the drugstore, but green food coloring is just as good—you can buy it in any grocery store or supermarket. Dip a small cotton swab in the jar of coloring and brush the bright green color across the top of your teeth on the gum line, and into the cracks between the teeth. The plaque will take the stain (clean tissue and tooth enamel will not), so you can see just where it is hiding. With a very soft toothbrush—this is the one time that nylon is better than natural bristles—brush away all the stained material. Rinse and brush again until it is all gone.

An important way of clearing bacterial deposits from tooth surfaces is to floss your teeth once a day. Here is the correct way to floss:

1. Use about 18 inches of waxed or unwaxed floss, or dental tape.
2. Hold the floss between your thumb and two fingers of each hand. This will give you control of the floss movement. Work the floss entirely through the small cracks between the teeth. Work back and forth several times.
3. Don't skip any teeth. Work on the front teeth as well as the sides and back. Some teeth will require going over several times.
4. For the bottom row hold the floss between the two fingers and thumbs as before, and push with a strong downward motion. Try not to pull the lips out of shape unnecessarily.
5. After flossing each crevice, pull the floss all the way through the hole, dropping one end of the floss. Never try to pull the floss from the gums to the edge of the teeth; it will weaken fillings and caps.
6. Rinse the mouth after flossing every few teeth to rid your mouth of the debris that you have loosened from your teeth and gums.

After flossing, brush your teeth well to keep them smooth and polished. When brushing, don't forget a final brushing of the tongue.

Avoid between-meal snacks. The fewer food contacts you have, the less chance plaque has to form: bacteria live on the food residue. Try not to eat, drink, suck, or chew any gum or liquid that might have sugar in it; this includes alcoholic beverages. And brush often, going up and down the tooth—not across.

Here are some easy, inexpensive cleaners and brighteners for your teeth that you can make at home:

LEMON RUB

1 small strip of lemon rind

Rub the strip across the teeth and gums. It will remove brown stains from your teeth, and slightly bleach darkened teeth. But be sure you rinse well. The lemon is acid, and left on the teeth it can affect the enamel. You can substitute pineapple, tomato, apple, or other slightly acidic fruits for the lemon. But, again, remember to rinse well. Pineapple juice and strawberry pulp are reported to be the best tooth-whiteners.

TOOTHPASTE

1 tablespoon kosher salt	3 tablespoons glycerin
3 tablespoons baking soda	

Mix together in a shallow wide-mouthed jar that can be covered and kept in the medicine chest. Add your favorite flavoring if desired. This recipe makes about the same amount as in a tube of commercial toothpaste; use it sparingly.

After each brushing massage your gums with your finger, and exercise them often, prodding your gums just at the point where they meet the tooth with rubber stimulators, or very soft wooden toothpicks.

Best Brows

The shape of your eyebrows affects all of the contours of your face. Eyebrows are as distinctive as lips, nose, or eyes—they act as signals. One small movement of your brows can convey a thought or emotion as clearly as any speech.

Heavy brows—from Joan Crawford's to Brooke Shield's style—can balance a strong or angular jaw. Delicate or arched brows can give a come-hither look to small or deep-set eyes. The natural arch of the eyebrow usually follows the bone structure under the skin, growing along the curved eye socket. It is entirely normal to have stray hairs both above and below the eyebrows.

There is no "perfect" shape for brows. They can only be perfect when they are in balance with your other features. Everyone's brows are unique, so keep your brows as natural as possible, shaping them only to enhance your other features. A few shaping tips:

- Your brows should begin over the inside corner of the eye. If your eyes are too close together, begin your brows slightly inside the white; if your eyes are very wide-set, you can allow the brows to almost meet. (The ideal distance between your eyes is one eye-length.)
- The highest point of the brow—the arch—should be directly over the outer edge of the iris. If you want to effect a wider look across the eyes, keep the brows looking open by moving the highest point of the brow to over the outer edge of the eye.
- To find the point where the brow should end, draw an imaginary line from the outer corner of the mouth to the outer corner of the eye, and then extend that line upward. The point at which it hits the brow is where the brow should end. If you have a narrow face and want to broaden the brow area, however, extend the brow slightly, but be sure that there is at least one eye-length between the end of the brow and the hairline.
- Check your brows. Are they at the same level? They should be, but usually there is a slight difference. Adjust that difference with a pencil or a tiny sable paintbrush, or an eyeliner brush that can recreate missing hairs and cover up sparse spots.

When filling in your eyebrows with makeup, use at least two different shades of pencil/liquid unless your hair is black, and work with short, light, even strokes. Try to imitate an actual hair:

Hair Color	Brow Color	Pencil/Liquid Brow Makeup
blond	blond/honey	ash blond, gray, beige
ash blond	blond/ash blond	platinum, gray, brown
brown/dark brown	brown/ dark brown	black, gray, brown
black	dark brown/ black	gray, dark brown
auburn	honey/rust	brown, gray, rust

Tweezing overgrown brows can seem to change the shape of your eyes. But over-tweezing is a common mistake and to avoid getting carried away, tweeze under the brow, not above the brow. For perfect and painless tweezing you'll need:

- warm water
- antiseptic (witch hazel works well)
- cotton
- oil (castor oil is best for eye area)
- tissues
- eyebrow brush
- tweezers (Good tools are always best. Tweezers come in different shaped tips; using one that's pointed, slanted, or straight-edged is a matter of personal choice. There are even some new styles that combine a tweezer with a small battery light.)

Start on the hairs between the brows, because this area is less sensitive than under the brows. Soften the brows by placing cotton saturated with hot water over the brows for a few minutes before tweezing. The warm water will soften and relax the skin, making the tweezing easier and pain-free. (If there is discomfort, you can use an anesthetic gel; try a product used for teething pain.)

Grasp each hair at its root, not at its end, with the tweezers and firmly pluck in the direction of the hair growth. Sponge the tweezed area frequently with warm water, followed by a dab of antiseptic lotion, such as witch hazel. Finally, rinse with cool water to close pores.

If you are bothered by a low hairline or a fine spray of hairs over your brows, waxing is a way to eliminate these hairs for about four weeks. The tweezed area will have to be checked for regrowth about once a week, because many hairs are dormant and will not be visible at any one tweezing.

How Your Brows Can Reshape Your Face

Problem	Solution
Low Hairline	A low, smooth, almost horizontal brow will give more height to forehead. Use a light color foundation on forehead.
High Forehead	Arch brows slightly to detract from the open forehead. Use deeper foundation on the forehead. Break forehead with soft wisps of hair.
Wide-set Eyes	Extend the brow line slightly between the eyes.

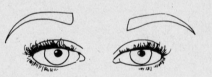

Problem	Solution
Close-set Eyes	Make eyes appear farther apart by widening the distance between the brows; draw attention to the outer edges of the brows by extending them slightly.

Problem	Solution
Round, Full Face	Keep brows short; arch the brows as high as seems possible at the peak, and keep brow ends up.
Narrow or Long Face	Create a horizontal line across the face by keeping brow peaks flat. Taper the ends slightly for a delicate, graceful look.
Narrow Brow, Wide Jaw	Arch brows slightly at ends. Begin the brows at the inside corners of the eyes, and keep the line smooth.

Problem	Solution

Square, Angular Face Create a high arch in the middle of each brow. Keep the brow peak smooth and curved.

Removing Eye Makeup

Because the skin on the eyelids, under the eyes, and on the temples is so thin, it seems to show age first. This early wrinkling can be hastened by rough treatment—and by stripping the natural oils of the skin when you take off your eye makeup. The goal is to remove all of the color without using so much that it gets into your eyes, and without rubbing the skin so that it is stretched and weakened.

Most eye makeup removers rely on mineral oil for dissolving the shadows and liner oils and waxes, and to help float away the pigments. There are also nonoil-based removers; they are solutions of water and boric acid or glycerin which allow you to reapply makeup immediately. This kind of remover can be very harsh and drying. The best routine for your skin seems to be a combination of both oily and nonoily removers. Use an oily remover first, and then follow with a nonoily remover if you want to reapply your makeup. Reverse the order if you're going to bed.

Oily or nonoily, apply the cleanser with absorbent cotton and a very gentle touch. Use two or three applications until the cotton comes away clean. If the skin is loose and sagging, support it with one hand as you use the other hand to wipe away the color.

To cleanse your eye area without stretching or pulling the skin, or damaging the underlying connective tissue in any way, you'll need cotton swabs, a tissue, and oil. Castor oil is excellent for this cleansing because any oil left on the lashes or brows will leave your lashes glossy and thicker.

Place a tissue under the eyelashes, and dip a cotton swab into the oil. Close your eye; gently work the swab of cotton from the base of the lashes to the tip, so that the oil carries the color onto the tissue. With another swab, paint a coating of oil over any eye shadow that might be between your lashes and your eyebrows. Using the tissue, blot the oil and color off the upper lids and the brow bone. As you blot, press the fingers gently against the tissue, so that the oil-soaked and loosened color is absorbed into the fibers of the tissue. Work from the outer eye toward the nose. Work gently—oiling and blotting—until all of the color is gone. Then, blot carefully so that excess oil doesn't get into your eyes.

Use a clean tissue for the final blotting. The gentle tapping with your fingertips as you blot will stimulate the orbicular muscles of the eyelids.

Puffs, Circles and Bags

The skin of the eye is very thin, and it seems to age before any other skin on the face. This causes small, unpleasant little lines and marks around your eyes. Bags develop because as you age the fat pads that protects the eyeball shrink and the little deposits of fat work their way past muscles and membranes to lodge just under the skin in the lower lids. Very little can be done to prevent this from happening because the size of your eye socket is predetermined by heredity, as is the thinning of the skin and fat pads.

You can make the bags less noticeable by using a highlighter under the bag, and a slight shadow just at the middle of the protruding little sack. Be very careful when you dot the colors together to blend them; it is easy to smudge the highlight on to the bag, and make it look even worse.

Puffy eyes come from an accumulation of fluids in the eye area: too much sleep, too little sleep, a cold, an allergy, or even sleeping on your face can produce this sort of bleary-eyed look. If you find that you are often bothered, raise the head of your bed with small blocks so that your head is actually higher than your feet. This often helps. Cool, moist tea bags, cucumbers, and grated-potato compresses also help. Many women find that cold milk compresses work well, and yogurt works for some, too. If the puffs are an allergic reaction or due to a cold over-the-counter antihistamines often work well.

Circles and dark skin under your eyes appear when you're tired and pale. You've probably had dark areas all the time, but when the rest of your face is very pale, or your nutrition isn't right, or you have anemia, these dark areas are more visible. You can avoid these circles by avoiding stress (yes, stress creates melanin, the coloring substance of the skin), wearing dark glasses when you're out in the sun, and eating a diet rich in iron.

Cosmetic camouflage can be achieved by using deep, intense colors in your eye shadows that are over the eyes, and using mascara only on the upper lashes to distract attention from the lower lids.

Eyeglasses

More than half of all American women wear corrective glasses, and sunglasses are one of the most popular fashion accessories. Glasses help you to see better—and also can make you look better. When selecting glasses you have the choice of frame and lens color and shape, within the current fashion or style. Makeup experts usually advise wearers to choose frames that will contrast with the shape of their own face.

Shape   The general shape should contrast with the shape of your jawline or facial proportions. An angular or squarish face needs rounded or curved frames; a long or pointed face needs strong horizontal lines across the brow or bottom of the glasses frames.

   The frames should be wide enough to balance the length of the face—about half as wide as it is long. If your face is very wide, be sure the frames do not extend much beyond the outer corner of the eyes.

Eyebrows   The top edge of the frames should cover the eyebrows and blend with them. If the eyebrows appear over the tops, this double set of horizontal lines can make the chin look weak.

Nose   If your nose is long, choose a frame with a low bridge that will cut across the middle of your nose. A short nose will appear longer if the glasses bridge is high.

Eyes   Close-set eyes appear wider apart if the bridge piece of the frames is clear and straight. Wide-set eyes can wear frames in which there is a very narrow bridge.

   The color or the finish of the frame should be geared to hair and skin color, or contrast with it. Generally the lighter the hair, the lighter the frame color. Bright, clear "jelly-bean" colors seem to make the eyes look younger and clearer.

   Pink, rosy, or purple shades can make a sallow skin look healthier. Blues, greens, and grays tone down ruddy or blotchy skins.

   Tinted lenses, according to Dr. Margaret Dowaliby, let through about 80 percent of the available light, and are cosmetic rather than functional. Real "sunglasses" must block about 75 to 90 percent of the available light. Medium-gray or green lenses are best for sunglasses because they distort natural colors the least.

Some do's and dont's of glasses wear are:

- Do select frames with an upward tilt; they seem to lift an older face.
- Don't use lash-lengthening mascara if you wear glasses with plastic lenses—it tends to scratch the plastic.
- Do use a 3-way mirror to check on side and three-quarter views of any frame you are considering.
- Do wear eye makeup under your glasses; especially if you are near sighted. Lenses for myopia make the eyes look smaller.
- Don't forget to protect the skin around your eyes on cold windy days by wearing clear glasses. They are also a great dust barrier.

All Day, No-Fade Makeup

If you leave the house looking great but find that makeup is melting, bleeding, feathering, and fading by noon, you're not alone. There are many solutions to the problem of keeping your "powder dry" (but not caked) and your foundation and colorants moist, but few of them are practical for busy women who work or travel. The following makeup and the step-by-step techniques are adapted from a demonstration given by Françoise Ramage-Delpuch, a French aesthetician. They work—you can extend your makeup life from 4 hours to more than 12 hours by following these simple procedures.

Moisturizer Start with a moist, but not dripping, face. Apply a very thin but even coat of moisturizer with sweeping strokes. The moisturizer should vanish on the skin, leaving it soft but free of any waxy feeling.

Foundation Dot the foundations on your skin, using a lighter tone in shadowed areas, a darker tone where you want to diminish fullness.

Using a damp cosmetic sponge, lightly pat the foundation, spreading it evenly in a very thin layer over the entire face. Carefully blend the foundation over neck, cheeks, under the tip of the nose, forehead, inner corners of the eyes, and if your hairstyle permits, your ears. Dampen sponge with cool water and smooth again, adding a dab or two of make-up to cover blemishes or discolorations. This primer coat is basic for good results.

Sculpture   Using concealer or contour, you can now correct minor flaws and create the illusion of a perfect symmetrical face. Apply light concealer on the shadows under the eyes, and smooth and blend. The lighter tones will soften aging shadows. Thin the nostrils, erase the frown lines, and fill in diminished tissue.

Using a medium-brown contour pencil or brush, surround the upper lid to the brow bone, and apply under the brow bone to contour cheeks. Blend and smooth carefully. Use damp sponge dipped in water for pencil, a bit of cotton for a powder blush.

Powder   Dip a large, soft powder brush into the powder and place the amount needed in the palm of your other hand. Use your palm as a palette and stipple the powder into the foundation. The effect should be translucent. Brush off excess; dust the entire face with a clean, soft brush. Close eyes and powder the lower lids, holding the brush flat.

Eyebrows   Start the eye makeup with the brows. Using a soft, clean brush, shape the brows and free them from any lingering powder. With a soft pencil extend the brows slightly; peak brows at the outer edges of the iris to give a wide-eyed look. Shape brows to be parallel with the shape of the upper eyelid.

Eyeliner   Using a soft black pencil for brunettes, gray or dark brown for blondes, continue the curve of the eye. Start at about the middle of eyelid and move to the outer corner. On the lower lid, draw from the outer third to the edge. Form lines slightly beyond the outside edge to enclose a triangle of skin. With small brush, sponge, or fingertip, smudge both lines. Work carefully and slowly. The line should be bold near the lids and feathered outward. As you blend and smudge, be careful not to fill in the triangle at the outer edge of the eye.

Shadow   Now apply a neutral shadow, one that matches the color of your hair or of your dress. Gray and brown are best. Use the powder under the eyes, too, and then bring it out around the extended triangle. Blend the pencil and shadow carefully. Select a lighter shade—gold, pink, or a jade green and fill in the tiny triangle. The lighter color will open, enlarge, and extend the eye. Work the outer corner triangle, moving inward. Bring a lighter color just under the brow and blend it into the midrange colors.

Outline	Apply a line of black kohl close to the lashes. (It may close the eye slightly, but it will define the shape.) Apply a dot of bright pink shadow at the inner corner of the eye. Smudge colors and blend together.
Eyelashes	Brush mascara on upper lashes from roots to the tips. Apply mascara slowly and patiently. When applying mascara on the lower lashes, protect the shadow on the lower lid with some tissue under the lashes. Powder the lashes lightly and apply a second coat of mascara.
Blusher	Using a neutral brown or deep tan shade of blusher and a soft brush, apply the contour-blusher over the areas that were sculpted with a darker tone of foundation. Blend this blusher in the hollow under the cheekbone and over the brow bone toward the hairline. (Keeping the forehead slightly lighter than the face draws attention upward and elongates the face; if the forehead is slightly darker than the lower face, the jaw seems wider and fuller.) The contour blusher gives movement and animation to the face. Now a dusting of pink tone or gold-orange tone applied deftly over the brown bone for highlights. As a last touch apply a bit of pink or orange near the hairline and across the bridge of the nose. (*Note:* These makeup tips model the face in several ways: with foundation, concealer, contour, and blush. If you find that one method works best for you, you can use that technique alone, or in combination. The use of several techniques, however, prevents color fade-out.)
Lips	Foundation has been applied to the lips, and while you were using shadows and concealers the foundation has set; now powder lightly. Decide on the outline of the lips and select a pink-brown lip pencil for a natural look, or a pencil close to the color of your lipstick for a more polished look. Draw a letter "V" at the center of your top lip, opening the V for a wide-jawed look, closing it for a defined Cupid's bow. The beginning and the end of the letter should be no wider than the edge of each nostril. Use small pencil strokes to avoid an outlined look. Then, outline the rest of the upper lip as far as the corners of the mouth. Make all outline adjustments with your pencil—raise the lip corners, make lips fuller or thinner, and so on. Pay special attention to the curved Cupid's bow, aim for perfection. Check to be sure the upper and lower lips are symmetrical; if you need to make corrections, do them with a white pencil. Once the lips have been clearly outlined, powder lightly again, and using a clean lip brush, smudge the side of the pencil that is

Lips
(cont'd)

on the inside of the lip line. Continue smudging until the edges are clean, but the lip is slightly covered with pencil. Select a lipstick shade that harmonizes with the blusher. (You can blend gloss with the lipstick for easy application, but the lipstick will not be as long-lasting.) Keep your lip firmly against your teeth and follow the line just inside the pencil as you apply lipstick. Use steady, even strokes. If you lift the corners of your mouth with one finger, you can get a clear outline to the very ends of your mouth. To make lipstick last longer:

1. Blot freshly painted lipstick with tissue.
2. Dust blotted lips lightly with powder, being careful not to smear the powder or lipstick.
3. Carefully apply a second layer of lipstick.
4. Use your pencil to apply the final finishing touches.

After you've completed this makeup, check the color and balance in a well-lighted mirror or natural daylight. Make any blusher or color-balance corrections needed. Dust off any excess blusher or powder with a soft silk brush that is perfectly clean. Mist or spray the face very lightly with cool water. A plant sprayer or small perfume atomizer is pretty and works well.

Part of keeping your makeup fresh is remaining cool, calm, and unemotional. Stress can trigger glands that trigger hormone, and they trigger the oil glands. Oil, not water, mixes with the oils and pigments in your makeup and can make the colors change—or vanish. Your feelings can also flush or pale your skin—and change the temperature on the skin's surface. This will affect the life of your makeup.

Finding Your Best Makeup Colors

I'm a pushover for magazine advertisements. I always tear the pages out and rush to buy the newest colors. But I'm often disappointed. The lighting in drug- and department stores is artificial, and some of the most beautiful in-the-tube colors look ghoulish when applied. From foundation to eye shadow, mistakes are expensive—and depressing. What can you do with those not-quite-right colors?

First, don't hesitate to mix cosmetic colors. There is no reason not to combine products from different manufacturers, or mix two or more products or colors for a completely new look. The ability to combine, mix, dilute, smudge, blend, and thin are the skills of every makeup artist. And you make your own rules.

What are your best colors? No need to guess; go to the closet and look through the clothes you have. Chances are you've selected shades and tones that make you feel great and garner compliments. Of course, your color choices are somewhat affected by fashion—sometimes you may find yourself wearing a color just because it is popular. Then, consider your eye color; you can change your hair shade, skin tone can be darkened slightly with a tan or gel, but your eye color remains the same from a few days after birth through the rest of your life.

Study the chart below, and choose which color families might be best for you. Circle the color that appears most often in your own closet. You'll notice that your selections will probably tend to fall in one personality group.

Dramatic	*Conservative*	*Natural*	*Romantic*
Black	Blues	Khaki	Peach
White	Brown	Gold	Jade
Navy	Wine	Beige	Turquoise
Red	Pink	Forest	Shocking
Gray	Lavender	Green	Pink
		Camel	Cream

Now, circle the eye and hair color that is closest to your own natural shades.

Eye:	Black	Brown	Hazel	Green	Blue
Hair:	Black/ Gray	Brown	Honey/ Gold	Blond	Reddish/ Auburn
Skin:	Brown	Ivory/ Yellow	Pink/ Ruddy		

Skin tone can vary from light to dark, according to the amount and kind of coloring. A good way of checking your real skin tone is to look at the skin on the upper inside of your arm. It is rarely exposed to light and it is seldom tanned. It will tell you what your "born with" skin tone is.

The chart below is only a guide to the makeup colors that might best suit your coloring and your personality. Your own taste and skin color must be taken into account, so you must test and try every cosmetic to be sure that the shade or hue is suitable for you.

Before selecting any color, mix a small amount. You might be able to come close to your ideal colors by buying inexpensive cosmetics in the general tones you want, and then mixing them until you've created a completely personalized makeup for yourself.

	Dramatic	Conservative	Natural	Romantic
Eyes	Darker eyes are more able to balance a heavy, deep color. Keep tones vivid; blue or green mascara.	Use subtle, matte colors. Pick up a color near the face—blouse, scarf, pin, etc.	Keep colors in earth tones and natural colors. Avoid contrast shades.	Smudge all colors; use a very light touch.
Blusher/ Rouge	High color and clear tones—within the context of skin tone.	Color should be a deepening of general skin tone. Blend very carefully.	Try for an effect that is similar to how you look after a brisk walk or exercise.	Beware of fadeout with too-light or too-pink shades.
Lips	Bold lips of clear, strong color. Fuschia, wine, and even orange-reds suit you.	Corals, plums, and wines are soft, accepted colors.	Stains and lip gels will give you a natural look. Try browns and rust colors.	Blue-reds are making a comeback. Don't let yourself look drained with a too-light color.
Skin	To suit your dramatic personality select a matte foundation that plays up any unique coloring.	Bisque/beige works well in offices or where there are artificial lights. Warm up a too-pale skin.	Don't try to perfect skin with heavy covering. Play up healthy look and inner glow.	Set makeup with cool water. Strive for an even-toned look.
Hair	From black to platinum use a rinse to highlight sharp color tones.	Frosted highlights can blend colors and soften any harsh tones.	Shiny, flowing, soft texture of any color looks great.	Keep hairstyle soft and "touchable."

Mix Your Own Makeup

Foundation

- You can thin any foundation by mixing a bit with a few drops of water. Two very thin coats of foundation will give more coverage than one thick coat. (Thinning your own makeup also thins the preservatives, so add the water to a dab on your hand, not the jar.)
- Test your foundation color on your neck for color, and on your nose for wear-power.
- You can give your makeup a dramatic evening look by mixing a bit of pearlized eye shadow into the liquid.
- Black women who find their makeup looks pasty should mix a bit of warm-wine lip gel into the foundation.
- Liquid rouge mixed with your foundation can recreate or match a fresh tan look.
- If your foundation begins to look orange after a few hours, your skin's pH is not matched to the makeup. Apply the foundation to a water-moist skin to keep it on a neutral pH.

Powder

- Baby powder or cornstarch can be used for cosmetic powder. Scrape some powdered blusher in if you want a rosy, healthy look. Mix your own powder with baby talc for a delicate, feminine look.
- Mix powder into foundation for your own all-in-one touch-up or pressed powder. It eliminates chances of leaks and spills when traveling.
- Use lighter powder in areas you'd like to enlarge—darker powder to create shadows. Powder, as well as foundation and blush, can "sculpt" features.

Shadows and Liners

- Use pink lipstick as shadow—it is easy to control and will stay where it is put.
- Frost any shade simply by mixing it with a pearlized white. Glittery shadow can be made from an all-purpose gold shadow that can even be mixed with lip gloss.

- Make your shadow into a liner simply by wetting a fine eyeliner brush. With the wet brush, pick up color and rim the eyes.
- Set and enhance eye shadow color with a dab of petroleum jelly.
- Mix broken or unused cakes of shadow together for new color effects. Crush the cakes between sheets of paper, or in a sealed envelope. Mix together by shaking the envelope, and then pour into a shadow tray that has been "greased" with petroleum jelly. You'll have made a new shade. Here are some ideas:
    Smoky shadows: blues, gray, silvers, charcoals
    Muted earthy tones: greens, golds, umbers, browns, and beiges
    Floral looks: blues, pinks, purples, silvers
    Autumn fires: toasts, wines, browns, oranges, golds

Blush and Contour

- Deep, strong blushers make eye-opening shadows.
- Mix foundation with powder blush for a fade-free cream blusher.
- Turn a matte blusher into gala wear by adding a pearlized shadow or bit of powder.
- Mix powder and plum-brown shadow for a blusher.
- Mix lip color and petroleum jelly for a smooth cream blush.

Lip Color

- Using foundation and powder under lip color keeps it fresh hours longer.
- Mix lipstick and cream blusher to help colors coordinate.
- Brown-wine eye shadow can be used as lip stain when mixed with petroleum jelly.
- Blend several lipstick bottoms into a new lipstick by melting several colors together in an egg poacher. Mix the colors with a wooden toothpick until shades are blended. Make a tiny funnel of aluminum foil and pour into empty tubes or color pots.
- To tone down a garish or orange hue, mix with wine or berry.
- If your teeth are yellowish avoid orange-tone lipsticks; if they have a bluish cast, no blue-red lipsticks. For the whitest-looking teeth a clear red is best.

Nail Color

- Thin old polish by setting bottle in warm water, or add remover very slowly, a few drops at a time.
- Mix small amounts of different shades together in empty bottles. You can create a shade to match any outfit.

Match Your Makeup to Your Sport

Over half of all Americans exercise or participate in some active sports each day. Health clubs, dance groups, exercise classes, and other social meeting places are a great way to get to know people, and in some cities they are replacing singles' bars. Of course that means you'll have to look your best while exercising to look your best, and that isn't easy. A fantastic leotard and leg-warmers mean your makeup has to adapt to hot sticky gyms and wind-whipped tracks.

Cosmetics and exercise are compatible, if you follow a few basic rules. Makeup for outdoor events or the revealing lights of a gym is very different from makeup for the office or for evening wear. Find your sport, or the activity you favor, in the list below:

Running	Fast footwork means perspiration and dilated pores. Don't depend on products with an oil base if you're working out indoors or in warm weather. Your own oil glands will be stimulated and you'll be shiny enough.
Tennis	
Handball	For outdoors, remember a sunscreen. A water-based foundation with a high SPF (over 15, or even 20) is ideal. Use waterproof mascara, or have your lashes dyed. Brush brows with petroleum jelly to keep them glossy and in place. Emphasize your eyes by lining them in gray or dark brown pencil. Protect the skin around your eyes by dotting the area with oil or moisturizer. Dust brow, chin, and cheeks with a light blusher in peachy tones.
Racquetball	
Squash	If you're running or playing in warm weather, keep your cosmetics in the refrigerator and apply them to water-cooled skin, and they'll last through a marathon. Spray your skin with splashes of cool water whenever possible.
Paddleball	

Martial arts   These can be the most fun and the hardest work. The exercise will raise your body temperature and make your skin glow, although signs of stress will show in your expression—especially if you're a beginner.

Yoga

If you wear glasses, attach them to a pretty ribbon so they don't slip; if you wear contact lenses, it is best to remove them before exercising.

Aerobic dancing

Start with very clean skin and then spray with an acid mist or splash with cool water. Because many of these exercises/sports are done indoors, watch out for color-draining overhead lights. Use a light water-base foundation and a cream blush or a colored gel to give yourself a fresh, outdoor look. Spread the gel over the cheeks, nose, and into the hairline.

Jazz dancing

Use a toast or pink shadow on the eyes, or use a soft crayon to frame them; smudge and blend all the colors. Double coat your lashes and use a clear, bright lip gloss. Your face will shine, and lips should match the shimmer.

Calisthenics

If you use a sweatband, avoid using foundation on your forehead. The friction of the band will rub the makeup into your pores and encourage blemishes.

Weight training

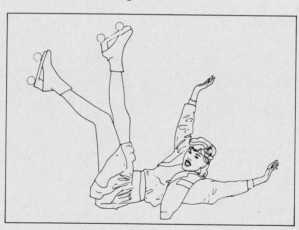

Swimming   Obviously this is the time for sunscreen and waterproof makeup, if you're enjoying outdoor water sports. If you limit your swimming to indoor pools, the sunscreen can be omitted.

Water polo   If you can't find waterproof makeup in your neighborhood, you can use a concealer thinned with oil. Blend it carefully on jaw and neck and be sure it matches shoulders.

Surfing   Powder blusher would vanish in the water, so use cream blusher, or a waterproof blusher.

Scuba diving   The shimmer of water means you need shadow; use a crayon or cream to protect your eyelids. A double coat of waterproof mascara will protect you from glare and frames your eyes as well. If you dot the inner corner of your eye with a pink pencil, the white will look clear and fresh.

Waterskiing   *Hand tip:* Smooth the backs of your hands with oily sunscreen; it will prevent some of the water wrinkles; and don't forget shoulders, insteps, and knees for the same protective treatment.

Wearing makeup for outdoor sports is good sense as well as good looks. The pigments act as a partial block against the sun's ultraviolet rays. Many cosmetics also include sunscreens.

After your energizing and relaxing workout or exercise you should shower as quickly as possible. Don't allow the oils from your own skin, mixed with the salt residue of perspiration, to cool on your skin; it will clog pores. Chlorine and other disinfectants are skin irritants, and if you're a pool swimmer, rinse off all the pool water as quickly as possible. Rinse your hair after swimming in a pool. Algicides containing copper compound interact with chlorine to produce a greenish hue on blonde or light hair.

If your skin is oily, you can enjoy the sauna, but if it is dry, you should cover your face with a protective vegetable oil. Sensitive skin can be stimulated by the sauna so much that small broken capillaries can appear after just a few sessions. And beware of cold water—pools or showers—after a session in the sauna. Let your skin cool slowly and naturally.

The steam room with its moist heat is kinder to your skin than the sauna. If you can, gently exfoliate your face, shoulders, arms, legs, and body with a few handfuls of granulated sugar as you steam. The sugar will seem to melt on your skin after a few minutes—just enough time to slough away the dead skin cells.

As soon as you leave either the steam, sauna, or warm after-exercise shower, slather your body with oil or a moisturizer. Use enough to cover your skin smoothly and pat it in, using gentle taps, slaps, and kneads. Then you're ready to apply a light coating of makeup, and face the world renewed.

6
Keep It Clean

The most recent skin-care theory involves taking it off, not putting it on. Since the introduction of commercial creams, the emphasis in skin care has been on the benefits that can come from applying unguents and packs, ointments and masks—on top of the skin. The hope had been that some of the effects of this surface treatment would seep down through the skin's surface to "penetrate" the skin.

We now have a different approach: Get off the old makeup, debris, dust, grime, oils, and pollution. Keep the skin smooth, sweet, and young by keeping it clean and encouraging your skin to renew itself.

Cream versus Soap

If there is one skin-beauty ritual that everyone must perform to look her best, it is washing. The secret of clear, beautiful skin begins with the complete removal of even the tiniest traces of dirt, oil, cosmetics, makeup, and your own cells as well as bacteria—at least twice a day: morning and night.

The old controversy between creams and soap has been complicated by the increased popularity of nonsoap cleansing bars and soft-soap creams. You'll have to be guided by your own preferences, but keep in mind that nonsoap beauty bars have most of the pluses of soap and few of the drawbacks.

Soaps were once made from fatty acids, and now are often a combination of natural products and synthetic detergents. They can be strong and harsh—highly alkaline and irritating—or they can be oily and mild.

The manufacturer's formula makes a great difference. Dove is one of the mildest commercial soaps.

The great advantages of a soap are that it lathers easily and cleans very quickly and effectively. The disadvantages are that it sometimes leaves dry or sensitive skin slightly irritated and flaky, because soap needs numerous rinses to make sure that no residue is left. Neutrogena, Dove, Aveeno, Basis, and Purpose all rinse easily, without leaving any residue.

Soft soaps or liquids are similar to bar soaps but incorporate more oils in their formulas. This means they are less drying. But they are also less cleansing. You have to move them more on the skin to work up a lather, which means there is more of a tendency to stretch the skin. They also leave an oily coating, because of the added moisturizers.

Cleansing bars do not lather as richly as soap, leave the skin almost residue-free.

Coat your face with a low alkaline vegetable oil that acts as a primary solvent for any dirt and makeup. Follow with water and a no-soap washing bar and many rinses for the best solution to the cleanest face.

If you've been using a cold cream or cream cleanser, you haven't been getting your skin "squeaky-clean" and you may be leaving a residue of cream, with a higher than 5.5 pH on your skin's surface. Another reason to steer clear of cold creams and other cleansers is that they are difficult to remove without wiping your skin, and each wipe has skin-stretch potential.

Precleansing—The Secret Step to Clean, Smooth Skin

Cleansing your skin of old makeup, dead cells, and pollution or particles is probably more important to your skin's care than any lotion or cream you could apply. "Taking it off" is often passed over too quickly or carelessly, and one important step that is usually overlooked is loosening and dissolving the dirt and debris to make cleansing more effective and less irritating. Fast cleansing is important because wet skin is weaker and more subject to irritations than dry skin. Just as oil repels water, the oil in old makeup and your own sebum repels the water when you wash. The first step in getting your skin clean should be applying a dissolving oil.

A light oil such as sesame oil, corn oil, or even mineral oil can be used to dissolve and float away dirt and makeup pigments. Use a light touch; apply with no moving or stretching of the skin.

After applying the oil, cover your face with one of the layers of a two-layer tissue. Press the tissue onto the skin—do not wipe it across your skin; you are blotting, not blending! Peel the soiled tissue away. Repeat the procedure until the tissue comes away oily but makeup-free.

After precleansing, you are ready for the most important of all skin-care treatments—washing your face.

Wash Your Face

Most of us learned to wash our faces when we were very young. At that time most of us didn't worry much about wrinkles or sagging skin, and we got into some bad habits. Some of those habits stay with us all our lives.

Face-washing Equipment: Because you'll be washing your face often, and because it is important that you have a simple, easy-to-follow ritual so you will follow it consistently, it is sensible to set up the equipment you need to wash, and have it ready. You'll need:

1 bar of low pH soap, any mild soap, or a nonsoap bar.

1 jar of lemon and water mixture; a glass pint jar works well.

1 small sea sponge; the natural sea sponges wash easily and quickly.

1 jar of vegetable oil; use only a small jar and keep any additional oil in the refrigerator.

1 wide-necked sugar jar, or a basket full of paper-wrapped 1-teaspoon sugars.

Washing your face is the one thing you do—every day, usually twice a day, and sometimes more often. It is your most consistent beauty routine, and can affect your complexion adversely, or benefit it greatly, and yet, most women cannot remember exactly what they do when they wash. It is just that automatic! There are right ways to wash, and wrong ways. You can change the wrong ways in just a few weeks, even if you've been doing them for over 30 or 40 years. Here is the right way to wash up!

Stage 1   Start with warm water; wet your hands and carefully wash them with a gentle, mild nonsoap bar, or use a soap that has a pH of 4.5 or 5. Be sure your hands and nails are clean before touching your face. Rinse your hands well.

Stage 2   If your face needs to be washed to rid it of stale makeup, or the grime of the day, you should soften and dissolve the makeup so that you don't have to scrub your face to get the foreign matter off. Your old makeup can easily be dissolved with just a coat of vegetable oil—sesame oil, corn oil, olive oil, or peanut oil will work. Spread the oil over your face and throat. Blot or pat excess oil away with a tissue.

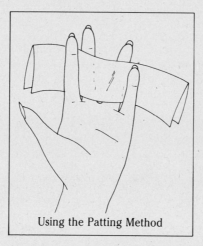

Using the Patting Method

Stage 3   A residue of oil will be left on your face after the blotting. Use a low pH soap or a nonsoap bar to wash away the residue of the oil and the makeup. The soap you use is not as important as how well you rid your face of the soap-scum and debris that the soap creates. Rinse, rinse, rinse. Make sure you wash away the residue. Now you're ready to free the new young skin cells that are waiting to be born.

Stage 4   Pour about a teaspoon of vegetable oil in the palm of your hand. With the other hand's fingertips, smooth the oil on your face. You can use upward strokes if you want, but more important than directional strokes, be sure that you're not moving your skin—simply spread the oil thickly over your skin, and around the eyes. Be very careful not to get oil in your eyes.

Stage 5   Pour about one teaspoon of sugar into the palm of your hand; it will mix with the remaining oil in that palm. Now spread the sugar over your oil-slicked face. The oil will make the sugar adhere to the skin. Using the fingertips and a very light circular motion, gently rub the sugar across your face. Pay special attention to the areas that tend to blemish or shine, or have large

Stage 5
(cont'd)   pores. Gently rub a bit of the sugar on the sides and tip of your nose. Do not use the sugar on the eye area, but it can and should be used on the throat and the mouth area. Do not spend more than a half-minute rubbing the sugar on your face. You want to free the dead cells, not damage the under-skin.

Stage 6   Rinse your face at least three times in warm to tepid water, add hot water, and a few more rinses. The sugar will immediately dissolve in the water, and the hot water will wash away the oil. If your face feels oily, or if you have a tendency to become oily, rinse again. Finish with cool rinses.

Stage 7   Do not dry your face. Any drying requires a movement of the face, and that—repeated at least twice a day—has a tendency to stress the skin. Drying also robs the skin of needed moisture. If you find your face too drippy, blot slightly under the chin. Try not to touch the eye area—you need the moisture there.

Stage 8   Soak a sponge (I prefer a sea sponge) in a mixture of lemon juice and water. Use 1 part lemon juice to 10 parts tap water. Pat the face with this mixture. It will make the skin smooth and blemish-free, and reinforces the slightly acid surface of the skin. (The sponge is easier to control than the popular spray, but this mixture works just as well in a spray bottle.)

You're now ready to apply a moisturizer, or a mixture of vegetable oil, mineral oil, and water that will protect the newly revealed cells from evaporation and the ravages of the elements.

Wash your face using this new technique at least twice daily. If you find your face reddened because of the abrasion of the sugar crystals, then stop for a day or two, and start again. Or, confine the use of the sugar crystals to once a day only.

Sugar-Cleaner

Sugar is a no-no when taken internally; so stay away from the sweets, and cut down on the sugar in your tea or coffee. But sugar, used as part of a cleansing program, can be one of your skin's best friends. When sugar melts it releases sucrose esters which dissolve oil, dirt, makeup, and accumulations of dead skin cells that can clog pores, or remain on the skin, making it look sallow and rough. Suzanne Hershfield, a California cosmetic chemist, who originated Product Organica (429 Nob Hill Drive, Walnut Creek, California), believes that the secret to clear blemish-free skin is actually to apply sugar to the skin. She thinks it might be the ultimate cure for troubled or acned skin.

Here is one of the ways Suzanne uses sugar for skin-cleansing and clearing:

Take ½ teaspoon of plain sugar and mix with a water-soluble cleanser, working it into the skin until it melts into a liquid. Mix with a no-alcohol or low alcohol water-soluble cleanser. Rub very gently, all over the face, but concentrate on oily or blemished areas. Rinse well with hot water, then warm water, then cool water, and finish with a splash of cold water. Use this scrub twice a week until the skin clears, and then once a week. If you have dry skin, use once a week. (If you buy sugar in the small individual packets that are used in restaurants, you'll find that you have just the right amount of sugar for one skin-cleansing treatment.)

Unlike many skin-care authorities, Suzanne Hershfield believes that you need only one moisturizer. She says, "What is important is the amount you use, and how often you use it. If you have greasy skin you may need to use a moisturizer only once a week." Here are several of Suzanne's home-made ideas:

BUTTER-UP

1 stick unsalted butter   1 ounce unsaturated oil
                                 such as almond oil

Blend together, and keep in the refrigerator. It will work as well as most commercial moisturizers.

SUZANNE'S SPLASH-MASK

1 orange   1 grapefruit
1 lemon

Prick the rinds all over the fruit with a fork. Peel the fruit, layer the peelings in a bowl, and pour water over the peelings. Cover the peelings with the water. Leave for two days; drain the water from the peelings, and use as a rinse.

SUZANNE'S CLEANSER

For the face: yogurt and bran, a spoonful of each. Work together, and rinse away, just as you would a soap.

Skin Balance (Acid/Alkaline)

During the past few years cosmetic manufacturers have become increasingly aware of the importance of matching the acid/alkaline balance of their products with the skin's natural acid/alkaline balance. Very often soaps, shampoos, and toners advertise that the product has a "low pH." It shows they have made an effort to preserve the natural acidic surface of the skin.

The acid/alkaline balance is measured in terms of the pH (potential hydrogen) of a product. An acid substance is capable of preserving organic substances. An alkaline substance is strongly caustic or corrosive to organic substances. A pH reading of 7.0 is considered neutral; the scale of measurement runs between 0, the most acid, and 14, the most alkaline. Most hair products are alkaline, and that is why it is so important that they are neutralized with an acid compound that will protect the hair from damage. For example, cold wave solutions are up to 9.6 on the pH scale, and soaps can also be as high as 9 on the pH scale. The most alkaline products used in cosmetics are hair depilatories that are usually above 10 on the pH scale—and are capable of weakening and dissolving hair.

Acids can be identified because they usually have a sour taste; some examples are lemon juice, vinegar, and citric acid. They contain hydrogen and a nonmetallic substance such as sulfur. Alkalines are usually bitter-tasting, soapy, and contain a metal, such as potassium.

How does pH affect cosmetic preparations and your skin? The skin and the hair are naturally slightly acidic. This natural acidity is helpful in retaining moisture and in controlling the microbes that can lead to infections. Most of these microbes don't thrive in an acid environment. (This is the reason that vinegar, a very acid substance, is so useful in preserving pickles and other vegetables; meats can also be partially preserved in acid brines.) Soaps, which are alkaline, act to dissolve and destroy skin particles and are also antibacterial. But the problem is alkaline substances don't distinguish between the bacteria and dead cells and your live skin. Excessive use of alkaline products can be very irritating to your skin. Ammonia is an example of an alkaline cleaner.

Dr. Irwin Lubowe and Barbara Huss, in their book *A Teen-age Guide to Healthy Skin and Hair* (Third Ed., New York: Dutton, 1979), say that the carbon dioxide given off by the skin combines with perspiration and amino acids of the skin to form an "acid mantle" covering on the surface. This acid coating helps to ward off infections. However, he says that frequent washing with soaps and the use of alkaline detergents can damage this protective surface.

Greg J. Story, a microscopist with Jhirmack, goes even further. He has stated that since the skin surface has been measured and found to be in the range of pH 4.5 to 5.5, the application of a cosmetic or lotion that is of a higher pH can cause skin irritation; a cosmetic will change color, and a lotion be less effective. The most common cause of lipsticks changing color after it is applied to the lips, and of makeup foundation turning orange, is that the pH of the cosmetic is different from the natural pH of the wearer's skin.

Story goes on to say that if a skin-care product is causing dry, flaky skin or irritation, the pH may be too high. A cosmetic that is well matched to the balance of your skin should leave it looking and feeling smooth, with no flakiness or redness.

How can you know, for sure, if your skin's vital "acid mantle" is intact or if some of your skin problems are due to constant irritation from alkaline substances? The best way is to test the pH of everything that touches your face or body skin. You can do this with Nitrazine litmus paper, available at most pharmacies. Your skin surface must be moistened before the paper is placed on its surface because the paper responds best to a liquid. Water, a neutral (pH of 7) substance, can be used to wet the skin. Using the Nitrazine paper for testing, makeup should have a pH of about 5 and skin-care products such as moisturizers and hand lotions should be approximately pH 4.5 to 5.5.

Of course your own natural pH will vary from time to time according to your life-style and your diet, your drinking habits, and even the medications that you might take. A woman's skin tends to be less acid just before menstruation—causing those irritating monthly acne flare-ups. Older skin also tends to be more alkaline, and have a higher pH than younger skin. This makes the skin sensitive, rough, and blotchy-looking.

The reason that mayonnaise is such an excellent skin-care substance is that it recreates the acidic surface of the skin. It combines the proteins of egg yolks (keratinized skin cells), the polyunsaturated oil (skin's oil), and lemon juice—an acidic substance that counters microbes and helps reinforce the skin's acid mantle. Mayonnaise is not the only substance that is pH-right for your skin. Try these acidic masks to rejuvenate and calm aging, irritated skin.

SKIN SANDWICH

Soften ½ stick of margarine. Mix with 2 tablespoons tomato juice. Spread the substance over two slices of very soft white bread. Apply the bread to the skin, and relax for about 10 minutes. Remove the bread, and rinse skin with warm water.

DRESSING UP

1 small egg yolk
2 tablespoons vegetable oil

1 teaspoon apple cider vinegar

Mix ingredients together and apply to the face. If necessary, cover your face with a water-moistened sheet of gauze, or a clean white cotton handkerchief. Allow the mask to remain on the face for about 10 minutes. Wash away with warm water.

The pH of the skin is lower on the surface of the epidermis than it is in the dermis layer. The dermis and under-layers of tissue are fed by the bloodstream. Blood has a pH of 7.4, which is almost neutral. This difference in the pH of the skin's outer layers and inner layers helps to reject foreign substances, and forms a natural chemical barrier.

What happens to the skin whenever a high pH substance, such as soap, is used on the skin? The skin acts immediately to protect itself, and to reproduce an oily, acid surface. The action of the skin to recreate the protective surface makes the skin produce more oils and a thicker horny layer. It takes the skin anywhere from two to four hours after the surface has been destroyed to recreate its necessary acid environment. This process encourages the growth of new skin cells, and also the production of the natural skin oils, sebum.

The effect of irritation from an alkaline product, and the activity of the skin to reproduce its protection, causes the skin cells to work more rapidly. This effort is thought by some experts to make the skin vulnerable to microbe invasion. But there is also evidence that this rapid production of protective skin cells keeps the skin vibrant and youthfully firm. You can get the best effects from this pH disruption by sloughing away the old outer layers without using harsh alkaline substances. One of the best ways is to whisk away the old cells with granules of sugar. The sugar, when dissolved in water, has a pH of 5.2; perfect for the skin.

After exfoliating with sugar, your skin will be "naked" of old cells and will need a low pH moisturizer for protection while it is building up its own new cells. An excellent moisturizer can be made by mixing water, oil, and mineral oil with a few drops of vinegar, lemon juice, or grapefruit juice. Shake this mixture vigorously before each use.

The introduction of low pH beauty bars rather than soap for washing are a boon for keeping skin's pH at a low number. These beauty bars usually contain protein, acid, and a binder, and are nontoxic. Jhirmack, Lowila, and Aveeno are the brand names for three of these beauty bars. Although they are more expensive than soap, with proper care they last for several months, and will go far toward keeping your skin properly acidic. In addition to keeping out germs, the acid level of the outer layer of skin also helps to keep the skin firm and tight. You'll notice that your pores appear smaller, and your skin appears tighter and firmer when you have correctly matched your skin's cleanser and cosmetics with your skin's natural balance.

Dr. Tina Johnson of Wichita, Kansas, has been involved in research regarding the effect of the acid/alkaline balance on the total health of the individual. She believes that the human body functions ideally at a pH between 5.4 and 5.8 (an acid condition). She has concluded that a myriad of chronic and acute diseases are related to pH imbalance, and has developed a chart to demonstrate some of these adverse effects.

Effect of pH on Human Chemistry

	pH Scale	
	4	Danger
	4.5	Heart attack, muscle cramps, spasms,
Stress		constipation
	5	Dryness of skin, aches and pains,
Ideal	5.4	ideal for human biochemistry
	5.8	
Low-Stress	6.5	Poor digestion, gas, bloating
	7	Cramps, clammy skin, flushing, colds, flu, sluggishness
	8	Headache, nervous trauma, nausea, exhaustion
Hi-Stress	9	Dangerous

When the body's pH goes too high, it is an indication that the adrenal glands, which help to control the pH balance of the body, might not be functioning correctly. The best way to check the acidity of the body is to check the urine, which is a fluid taken from the blood by the kidney, and reveals an accurate pH reading. If you feel your body pH is imbalanced, Dr. Johnson has suggested these therapies:

Methods for Controlling pH Balance

When the Nitrazine tape or paper is yellow (too acid), do the following:

When the Nitrazine tape or paper is green or blue (too alkaline), do the following:

To Increase pH

Baths (select one)

1. A hot bath or hot shower
2. A hot mineral bath
3. Mustard bath of ½ cup dry mustard in warm water. Soak 10 minutes.
4. A warm bath for 15 minutes with 1 cup of baking soda.

To Reduce pH

Baths (select one)

1. A cool bath
2. A cold shower
3. Soak in a tub of warm or body-temperature water with 1 cup vinegar added to the water; soak 10 minutes.
4. A tub of tepid water with 2 cups Epsom salts added to the water; soak 10 to 15 minutes.

For more about Dr. Tina Johnson's ideas, you can write directly to her. She is the president of DermaTherapy International, and the director of a Beauty Clinic and Training Center. She is one of the many beauty experts who is concerned with the total health of their clients. You can also write for a guide to drinks to control pH balance. Write to DermaTherapy, 3335 Oakland, Wichita, Kansas 67218 for further information.

7

New Skin in 20 Days

If you want your skin to always look new, then you must make sure it always *is* new. New skin cells grow naturally, but they do need encouragement. The "New-Skin" program is based on two sound ideas:

1. Ridding the surface of the skin of old cells
2. Stimulating a vigorous blood supply in the skin to help new skin cells grow rapidly

Both these goals are accomplished through a system of skin "sanding," followed by gentle but firm pats and taps that flex the facial muscles and engorge the muscles and the skin with oxygen and nutrient-laden blood. The program forces the growth of new cells and provides the needed materials for insuring healthy, perfect new cells.

To Slow Down Aging, Speed Up Cell Production

Cell renewal, or the ability of the skin cells to develop and grow, has recently become one of the focuses in skin care. The idea is to speed up this cell turnover process that continues all our lives, but lags slightly as we age. If we can keep the renewal process at very much the same rate it was when we were in our twenties, then, in theory, our skin might look like the skin of a 20-year-old forever.

When we are young, new skin cells move rapidly to the surface, and when they die they quickly flake away and make room for new cells. With age, however, worn cells seem to linger on the surface of the skin—dead. These dead cells do not reflect light, look dull and yellowish, and feel rough. Many cosmetic researchers and dermatologists believe that if the cells don't slough off fast enough, on their own, removing them can not only help the skin to *look younger* but also to *become younger* because the skin is forced to work harder to produce new cells to cover the body.

There are two ways to rid the skin's surface of these dead cells: one is mechanical, with an action much like sandpaper, an abrasive that rids the skin's surface of bumps, blemishes, and rough spots. The other method is chemical, and it has very much the same effect as does paint or finish remover on a piece of old wood.

The mechanical way of gently scraping, rubbing, or buffing the dead skin cells away is usually done by washing with a complexion brush, cleansing grains, or a scrub with particles in it, or by using a specially developed rough-surfaced pad such as Buf-Puf. This process of ridding the skin of the upper layer of dead skin cells leaves the skin fresh, clean, and invigorated. It is called exfoliating, or sloughing the skin. They both mean the same thing. Many experts agree that this process can be helpful to the skin, and can actually speed up the production of new cells.

The chemical way to rid the skin of the dead cells is not new either, but there has been more recent experimentation in this method. The idea is to use a chemical that will loosen the dead cells so they can be washed away. The chemical substances dissolve the weak protein bonds that hold the dead cells to the surface and have recently been combined with soothing emollients, so that as the skin is sloughed off, a protective coating is left to insure the health of the new cells.

To rid your skin of these old cells on your own, at home, you can use any of several methods, or a combination of methods. Here are a few possibilities:

Rubbing Dead Cells Away

cleansing grains (crushed apricot pits)
abrasive sponges (Buf-Puf, or something similar made of synthetic
   fibers)
dried plants (loofahs, hemp, reeds)
horsehair mitts (woven mittens that are rough and washable)
natural brushes (most of them are goat or other animal hair)

Pulling Dead Cells Away

clay masks (the clay absorbs the oils and moisture on the skin, and
  the dead cells are carried along)
peel-off masks (a sticky substance painted on the skin that pulls
  away the dead cells as it is pulled off)
creams (the mildest to float dead cells away on a semiliquid flowing surface)
gels (similar to the peel-off masks, but gels remain tacky and do
  not harden)

Chemically Melting Dead Cells Away

papaya (juice, the pulp of the fruit, or the rind of the fruit)
resorcinol (irritates the skin and causes peeling)
salicylic acid (topically applied aspirin irritates the skin and causes
  peeling)

There are problems with each of these methods; if overused, the abrasive method can irritate the skin, and it is not suitable for very thin
skins, nor should it be done carelessly in an overzealous manner because it can break through the acid surface of the skin and expose the
tender new cells to drying and damage. Over-scrubbing can also result
in broken capillaries. This is especially true of thin, aged skin. Also, if
skin is allergic to any of the grains, abrasives, or pads that are used, it
can become seriously inflamed. Care and caution must be used when
this technique is employed.

Care must also be taken with skin that blemishes easily. Rubbing can
stimulate already overactive oil glands. Acne can be triggered by too
much exfoliating.

If the chemical cell-dissolvers are used, even more caution must be
exercised because the sensation of pain doesn't stop you from applying
the cream or preparation—until it is too late! Many people have found
that the new creams which "stimulate new cell growth" keep their
skins flaking at an ever-increasing rate, so that a once-smooth—if not
youthful—complexion is reduced to a flaky dry one that might look
worse than it did before the treatment.

Both techniques work because both irritate the skin slightly, and
when the skin is irritated cell production is more rapid. Old cells are
opaque and do not reflect light; they are packed together, and they give

the skin a dull appearance. New cells look smooth, are translucent, and are smooth to the touch. If the cells do not linger on the surface of the skin after they lose their inner moisture and flatten, then your skin will always be new and look smooth and dewy-moist.

To keep the skin looking great you'll have to be sure that you provide the new baby cells with nutrition, water, and oxygen. Rubbing off the old cells without making sure that your new cells have all the potential for healthy and complete growth is like sending all your winter clothes to a charity without making sure that you have something warm for the next cold day. Waking up your cells' metabolism means waking up a need for oxygen and nutrition—and the blood supply to feed the cells of the new skin.

Sugabrasion: A Faster Way to New Skin

There is an interesting relationship between the rate at which upper epidermis skin cells are sloughed away naturally, or worn away, or scraped away, and the rate at which new cells grow at the lowest levels of the epidermis: They are always the same. Therefore, if the cells slough off on the surface rapidly, new cells in the lower levels will grow more rapidly. In youth it takes the body about a day—24 hours—to replace the layer of upper epidermal cells. But as we get older the process slows and in old age it takes about two days. Slower cell renewal means we are "wearing our skin two days instead of one." Sugabrasion helps you always wear new, smooth skin.

What is the sugabrasion method of rejuvenating the skin?
It is a way of continually ridding the skin of the very top cells that are dry, rough, and dead. The skin is constantly growing new cells and renewing itself; this technique encourages the process and speeds the new cells to the surface. The rate of cell growth adjusts so that the density of the skin remains the same. So, the more upper cells removed, the more rapid the new cell growth.

How can sugar create these benefits?
The sugar granules whisk away and eliminate many of the surface problems such as uneven color, sun damage, and fine dry lines. The stimulation of the abrasion "revs up" a dull complexion, leaving the skin with a healthy glow. It also removes dirt and impurities and seems to minimize pores. The stimulation leads to strengthened elasticity be-

cause after each gentle treatment there is a new bouncy layer of skin cells on the surface.

Can sugabrasion help fight acne?
The daily peeling removes the bacteria-attracting debris that block pores. This discourages blemishes before there is a chance of pitting and scarring; it opens clogged oil passages. It is also easy to use and needs only a light touch so that the skin's oil glands are stimulated.

Who should use the sugabrasion system?
Sugabrasion will benefit every skin type. Sugar—a natural granular substance—is softened by the skin's own moisture and will dissolve after a few short moments. Sugar leaves the skin's natural pH undisturbed, and so even the most delicate and sensitive skins can benefit from the light, natural abrasive.

How long must I use the technique?
You should include sugabrasion of the skin as part of your daily grooming as long as you want to encourage the growth of new skin cells—all your life! But after the first three weeks (about 20 days) you can cut down the abrasion to every other, or every third, day. Of course you'll want to use it often if you want to look your best every day.

How long do the benefits last?
If you've used sugabrasion as part of your daily cleansing ritual, it will take several weeks until its benefits fade away. The cell renewal will slow down without the encouragement of sugabrasion.

How much time will this technique take?
If you're sugabrading your skin more than a minute a day, you're spending too much time. The best part of the technique is that it works the way your skin grows—day by day. Use the technique every day if you can, but remember, you want to whisk off the flattened dead cells, not damage the newer cells.

What, exactly, is the procedure?
After washing your face with a low alkaline soap or a no-soap bar, cover your face with a soothing acidic oil, such as olive oil. The oil will act as a medium for the sugar. It holds the sugar on the face, and prevents the skin from being scraped or scratched by the granules. Apply granulated

sugar (white or brown) to the skin, dotting it on nose, chin, cheeks, forehead, and throat. The sugar will adhere to the skin because of the oil.

Using the pads of the fingers, roll and "sand" the abrasive sugar granules across the surface of the skin. You don't need to press; the granules will do the job of loosening and freeing the old skin cells. Don't use sweeping motions; small circular motions that do not move or stretch the skin are best.

After about a half-minute the sugar will seem to dissolve and it will be time to wash away the oil, dissolved sugar, and dead cells. Use warm water and a very light coating of soap lather to wash the skin clean. Rinse at least a dozen times with fresh warm water to rid the skin of any possible alkaline residue.

You can use this technique in the morning without the presoaping. But in the evening or before going to bed, wash away the day's grime before applying the oil of your choice. Always use the abrasion before a facial mask or other treatment. The new cells that are exposed through sugabrasion will allow any treatment to be more effective.

Can the technique hurt or be harmful?
Pain and irritation are useful because they alert us that something is wrong. Using the sugabrasion method should not hurt or cause any discomfort. The sugar crystals will dissolve after a few moments, and the oil also acts to protect your skin. Sugar is a natural vegetable product that is created in almost all plants and animals.

How does this technique differ from other skin peels?
Chemical peels often irritate the skin's surface and sometimes the side effects are unattractive flaking or rough skin. Sugabrasion, a method of mechanical skin peeling, is easier to control, and so there are fewer chances of skin irritation. Also, there are no aftereffects because no alkaline substance is used.

Deep skin peeling in a doctor's office, or hospital, is a way of ridding the skin of its upper layer in a dramatic fashion. If chemicals are used, the upper layers are burned away; if a mechanical device, such as a surgically sterile wire brush is used, the skin is abraded, or scraped away.

Sugabrasion scrapes away the upper layer—a few cells at a time. It takes only *one* treatment to reveal a cleaner, newer skin, and about 20 days to see a dramatic change. The advantages of sugabrasion are these:

1. Sugar is a natural substance.
2. New sugar is used in each treatment; there is nothing to collect

dead cells or bacteria, and nothing that must be washed. The sugar is convenient, and what is not used just washes away.

3. Sugar granules dissolve before the technique can injure the skin.
4. Sugar is good for the skin, attracting moisture.
5. Massaging with sugar rids the surface of dry, opaque, and discolored or rough cells.
6. It is simple, inexpensive, and it works.

How will my face look after I use the treatment?
Right after a treatment—even your very first—you'll notice that your skin is softer, clearer, and rosier. The pores will seem smaller, and the tone will be more even.

Are there any drawbacks?
Because the upper layer of the skin is thinned, and the surface of the skin is smoother, the light seems to penetrate the skin, making the blood vessels of the skin more visible. The abrasion of the skin does not create more blood vessels, nor weaken the ones that you have, but it does give the skin a rosy glow. Using sugar prevents overstimulating the skin's blood supply because it dissolves so easily, but sugabrasion exposes new skin cells to the air and to damage before they are completely flat, which makes them vulnerable to dehydration.

What about the sun? Will I burn more easily?
It is never a good idea to expose your skin to sun damage. The new cells that are exposed by sugabrasion are especially vulnerable to dehydration; the cells will dry out very rapidly unless they are protected. Old cells are rough, and they actually deflect the sun's ultraviolet rays; new cells are much more vulnerable. Avoid the sun after sloughing your skin. If you rid skin of old cells and then oil or moisturize your skin, you're creating a smooth surface that will act as a lens for focusing the sun's damaging rays.

Are there any precautions I should take when I use sugabrasion?
Yes, you must protect the new cells, keeping them moist and soft. Sugabrasion unclogs pores, and so natural oils can flow freely, but you should also coat the newly exposed skin with a thin coating of oil and water, or a light commercial moisturizer. If you want to make your own moisturizer, simply mix ½ cup of light oil and ½ cup of water and a teaspoon of mineral oil in a small bottle and then shake together vigorously. Apply the oil and water liberally—it will seal in moisture and keep your skin soft.

Can anyone use the technique—anywhere?
Anyone over 13 can profit from the technique. Some areas of the face and body are thicker than others, and some skin cells naturally remain on the surface longer than others. You can selectively slough the nose, chin, and other areas more vigorously than the eyelids, which are very thin. But abrasion can rejuvenate and freshen any skin, even the skin around the eyes and the neck.

Skin cell renewal, encouraged by abrading the upper level of the epidermis, uses the body's natural process to make and keep the skin youthful. The process of new cell growth can be speeded up by as much as 30 percent using this technique.

Your skin is unique; there is even a difference between the skin on your cheeks and on your eyelids. You can give each part of your skin the sugabrasion it needs by using this chart as a guide to your daily beauty ritual. Adjust the information on the chart to match the skin on different parts of your face and body, as well as the weather and your day's activities.

Skin	Oil/Medium	Soap or Cleanser	Frequency	Pressure
Eye area	Crisco, margarine	Oil only	Once a week	Very light
Throat	Thick vegetable oil (e.g., avocado, oil)	Mild soap or oil	Twice a week	Very light
Upper lip	Vegetable oil	Mild soap or oil	Twice a week	Light
Forehead	Thin vegetable oil (e.g., safflower)	Beauty bar or low-alkaline soap	Every day	Firm
Cheeks and jaw	Vegetable oil	Beauty bar or low-alkaline soap	Every day	Firm
Nose	Vegetable oil	Mild soap, Dove, Neutrogena, e.g.	Every day	Firm
Chin	Water and oil	Mild cleanser or soap	Every day	Medium
Shoulders	Water	Ivory, Vel, or strong pure soap	Every day	Brisk
Back, Elbows, Feet	Water	Ivory, Vel, or strong pure soap	Every day	Brisk

Stimuslaps

Stimulating the skin through the use of pressure, stroking, and massage is one of the oldest methods of skin care, and is an ideal technique to use in conjunction with sugabrasion. To use the stimuslap techniques properly requires some knowledge of anatomy and physiology, but it is easy to master the techniques with very little practice.

Where it works: The stimuslaps need not be limited to one area of the body. Stimuslaps can improve circulation to the face and neck, but they work on most parts of the body, the legs, arms, feet, and hands, too. Here is a list of the areas that can be "treated":

1. Feet, arches, ankles with pats and taps
2. Calves, thighs, buttocks with slaps and hacks
3. Shoulders, neck, and scalp with hacks and pats
4. Face, neck, upper chest, shoulders with taps and pats
5. Hands and arms with pats and taps

The basic rules: Stimulating slaps should never be applied to cool or dry skin. Before patting or slapping, apply cream or oil to the skin. The best oil is a thick vegetable oil. The oil softens the skin, permits easier hand movements, and it helps prevent pulling or dragging of the skin. The oil also lubricates and softens the skin so that there is no danger of tissue damage. Do not use the stimuslap technique if you suffer from acne, or any infection of the skin, or if you have a tendency to broken capillaries.

The stimuslap technique requires a firm, sure touch. As you master the movements you'll also notice some other pluses! You will develop stronger, more flexible hands, arms, and shoulders.

Before touching your face or body with stimuslaps be sure that your hands are immaculately clean and soft. You must wash your hands and nails carefully and then apply a coat of hand cream or oil. Your nails should be smooth to prevent snagging the skin. Your wrists and fingers should be smooth and flexible. Don't wear rings—and certainly not a ring with a set stone that might scratch your skin. Your palms should be warm and dry.

Every stimuslap session combines one or more of the four basic movements: tap, pat, hack, and knead. Each movement is applied in a specific way. The results of the stimuslap movements will depend on the force, pressure, and direction of your hand motions as well as how long the session is.

Be aware that your skin is a living, delicate organ and should always be treated with care and discretion. Avoid overstimulating the skin and do not pat or tap, hack or knead any more than the number of times specified. If your skin feels tender or inflamed in any way, do not attempt any of the stimuslap motions. What your skin probably needs is some soothing calm—not additional stimulation.

When and How

There are times when "less is better" and you should avoid skin stimulation: if your skin is windburned, chapped, or sunburned. But there are times when skin stimulation can help rev up your blood circulation and bring a healthy glow to your face and sparkle to your eyes:

— if you feel stressed and anxious
— if you feel tired and haven't had enough sleep
— if you're not getting enough exercise
— if you have a headache or eyestrain
— if your work keeps you sitting for long periods of time

The position of the hands and the direction of the movement of the hands is very important in getting the most stimulation from the fewest number of stimuslaps. Always follow the direction or path of the muscles. The stimuslaps should excite the skin and encourage an increased blood supply to the muscles.

How to Use Stimuslaps

Lightly tapping and slapping the skin is a nonaging way of stimulating your skin and encouraging a vigorous blood supply to your facial muscles and your skin. It is ideally suited for daily stimulation because it is a massage technique that does not move the surface skin away from the underlying tissues and muscles. The light taps actually exert a firming effect and help increase the local blood supply. Here is exactly how it is done:

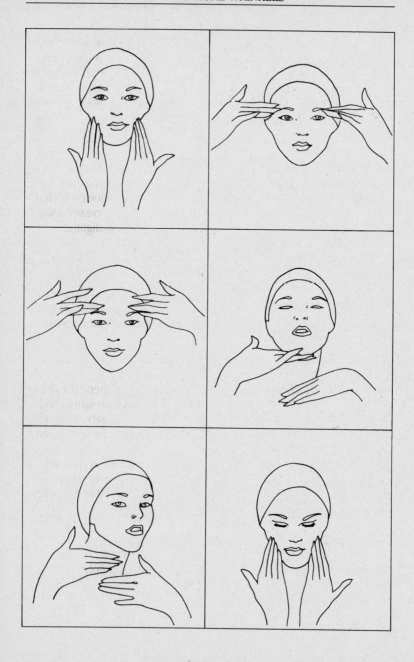

Taps

This motion is the most stimulating, but it must be done gently with care and restraint. In this form of skin stimulation only a light finger-tapping motion is used with the ring finger and the middle finger against the surface of the skin in rapid succession. The fingers must be flexible enough to create an even, light force over the skin, but also rigid enough to create a slight tingling sensation.

Pats

In the patting movements, the face is stimulated by the entire palm. Flexi-ble wrists allow the palms to contact the skin in light, firming, and rapid pats. Both hands can be used and each pat, which is not violent, nothing more than a light but firm momentary contact with the skin, creates a slight suction because of the oil on the skin, so the skin is lifted slightly.

Hacks

The gentle chopping motions made with the wrists and the heels (the outer edges) of the hands are excellent in stimulating the skin and under-muscles on the shoulders. Both palms and the fingers should be held slightly rigid. The sides of the hands should move against the skin in fast, light, alternating motions.

Kneads

This movement provides deeper stimulation than the others; it will im-prove circulation in the face and firm the jawline. The pressure should be light but firm. With the second knuckles of your fingers, press and roll in a kneading motion. The movement should be gentle and rhythmic—never jerky or violent.

Skillful stimuslaps affect your total well-being and your entire body—directly or indirectly. You will first notice a glow come to your facial skin; this is because of the increased circulation. But there are other, lasting benefits:

— soft and dense skin is encouraged
— fat deposits are reduced
— skin structures are nourished by greater blood supply
— glands within the skin are stimulated
— muscle fibers are firmed and strengthened
— nerves are soothed
— tension pains and muscle tightness are relieved

Although stimuslaps stimulate the skin, people find slow, light taps and pats very restful and relaxing. The faster the motions are the more invigorated you'll feel. Speed of the motions can be changed to suit your personal moods. If you want to use the pats as a wake-up, or as a mid-day stimulator, about a minute of rapid pats, taps, and kneads should do it.

As part of a complete program to keep your skin taut and youthful, the stimuslaps work best done for a very short period of time—about 1 minute to 1½ minutes—every night, before going to bed. Do not speed up the stimuslaps to get more in during that time; slow and steady firms the face, anything faster or harder will only be destructive.

Body Whisk

Anything that rids the surface of the skin of the dead cells can be called a "thinner" or exfoliator. But the surface of your body is so large that in order to use a method that is practical, it must be inexpensive, easy to apply, and fast-acting. Most people prefer rough grains or brushes that can whisk away the dead skin easily and quickly. Nina Walter, director of a beauty farm in Baden-Baden, West Germany, says that the thicker skin on the body can really benefit from the brisk scrubbing of a brush or an abrasive mitt. The masseuses in the exclusive spa use long, firm strokes on the arms and legs, back and body; they brush toward the heart, up the legs, and from fingers to shoulders on the arms. Try the following body peel; it will make you feel tingling clean and prepare your body for stimulated cell growth.

All you need is a half cup of kosher salt or sea salt, a half cup of bran or raw oatmeal (the oatmeal is better for very delicate skins; the bran works well on rough skins, arms, and feet), about two tablespoons of a whipped corn-oil margarine, and a warm bathroom.

Place a very large terry towel on the bottom of your bathtub. You'll have to sit there for about 20 minutes, and it makes the tub much more comfortable.

In a small bowl, mix the salt, bran or oatmeal, and the whipped margarine. (The mixture of the bran and salt recreates the nutrients and salts of seaweed.) Water can be added if the mixture becomes too doughlike; the consistency should be spreadable with your fingers.

Standing naked in your tub, and starting with the feet, gently apply the body-food on the surface of the skin. Work up the legs, and don't forget the skin on the upper thighs and buttocks. If you have trouble covering your back and shoulders, you may want to apply the concoction to a small hand towel and rub the towel across your back.

Don't forget the arms, elbows, shoulders, and breasts; but, do not rub the delicate skin on the nipples. Some people might even prefer to cover the nipples with petroleum jelly to protect them.

When the body has been completely covered, rub a bit of the bodyfood up the back of the neck.

Sit down in the bathtub, and gently rub the entire body with the slightly abrasive mixture. It will have a rather pleasant texture, and the salt will act as a mild exfoliant while the bran and corn oil nourish the skin.

Now relax. Just sit in the empty tub, think pleasant thoughts, file your nails, or listen to music. After about 10 minutes, wash the bodymask from your entire body by briskly showering. Use alternating warm and cool water.

You'll find your skin glistening, smooth, and elastic. The color will be even and the texture exquisite. A final splash of cold water on your breasts (a traditional French method of keeping the breasts firm) and a coat of cream on your shoulders and legs will leave you ready to wear your most daring low-cut evening dress, shortest shorts, or skimpiest bathing suit.

8

Creams and Coverings

Cosmetics and Makeups

In the Federal Food, Drug and Cosmetic Act of 1938 a cosmetic is defined as any substance that is "rubbed, poured, sprinkled or sprayed on
the human body for cleansing or altering the appearance." A cosmetic
does not affect the body's structure or function. Medicines are defined
as products that treat disease and alter the body's function.

As cosmetics become more and more sophisticated, and as they become more effective, the gap between cosmetics and medicines becomes smaller and smaller. There is no reason why any cosmetic or
makeup should not only beautify, but also improve, or at least protect,
the skin, hair, or nails. For legal reasons the distinction between drugs
and cosmetics is important. Drugs must be proven safe *and* effective before they are approved for public use. Cosmetics need only be proven
safe.

Probably the most widely used cosmetic is soap; toothpaste, shampoos, shaving products, and makeups follow. In the last hundred years
there has been more progress in the development of skin-protecting
cosmetics than in the last thousand. A great deal of the progress is due
to mineral oil, an inexpensive and almost allergy-free substance that
has an endless shelf life, and can easily be combined with other oils and
with pigments to create skin-care preparations that make you look
good—and also are beneficial to the skin.

Secrets of History—and Before

Perfumes and cosmetics are usually discussed together in ancient scriptures. In China, Greece, Rome, and in prehistoric Mesopotamia, both men and women wore cosmetics. The need for oils and herbs to make balms and ointments was one of the major reasons for commerce. The ancient Chinese used love charms of herbs that were worn on the body. Even today, in some parts of the world, most cosmetics are made in small quantities by local experts—herbalists or perfumers.

Here are two historical cosmetic recipes that were used in ancient times. They still work, although I've adapted them to work around ingredients that are not easily available. Most of us can't get a quantity of chewed betel nut, nor would we want to!

SKIN CREAM (Minoan)

gum of frankincense	oil
wax (probably bees-wax)	nuts, ground fine

Similar to a cleansing exfoliant for your skin

7-OIL CREAM (Cleopatra's Formula; adapted)

2 tablespoons each of:

safflower oil	mineral oil
sunflower oil	olive oil
peanut oil	sesame oil
avocado oil	

Mix with geranium leaves, and allow to remain in a dark place for about 2 weeks.

The Cosmetic Composition

Most cosmetics that coat and/or color the skin are made of only four or five basic ingredients. For example, a skin cream that is designed to keep the skin moist, and to prevent dehydration, would include the following:

- The essential component that acts as a barrier against the outside is an oil of some kind. It might be lanolin, an animal oil, or a vegetable oil, or a mineral oil, such as petroleum jelly.
- An ingredient that acts to soothe the skin, such as chamomile, or an astringent and antiseptic such as camphor.
- To keep the oils and the active ingredients fresh and pleasant a preservative is added. Methylparaben is one of the most popular of these preservatives. Without preservatives cosmetics would deteriorate and turn rancid in a few days.
- To keep the other ingredients even and smoothly suspended in a creamy texture, an emulsifier, such as gum tragacanth, is usually added. If the cosmetic is designed to be in stick form, such as lip balm, a color pencil, and so on, a wax or paraffin to thicken the concoction is added.
- Finally, to make sure the cosmetic has an attractive color (ever wonder why so many "cooling" lotions are blue or green?) an attractive colorant is added along with a perfume to make the cosmetic pleasant to use.

Most cosmetics contain a high percentage of water. In many skin lotions over half of the liquid is just water. The base of most creams and cosmetics is an emulsion made of a mixture of oil and water. If there is more water than oil, then the oil is suspended in the water; if there is more oil than water, then the water is suspended in the oil; and if there is about an equal amount, they mix together evenly.

The more water that is suspended in a cosmetic, the better it is for your skin; but the faster the effects of the cosmetic vanish because of the evaporation of the water. The ideal cosmetics have just enough oil to replace any oil not produced by your own glands. And the oil should keep the skin at the same acidic balance as your own skin oils would. The color should be even if the cosmetic is a makeup, and the consistency should be easy to work with.

Creams

A trip to any drug-, department, or variety store will probably give you more of a selection of creams than you really need. There are thousands of creams on the market: some are white, some colored, some perfumed, some thick, some thin, some sticky, some smooth . . . and all of them are actually quite similar. They're all variations of a basic formula that is similar to cold cream. If the cream is meant to be left on the skin—as an eye cream or a moisturizer—then the cream is formulated to be less greasy than cold cream. If it is to be used as cold cream to carry away old makeup and debris from the skin, then it is quite greasy, and must be tissued or washed off.

The basic formula is often something like this:

stearic acid	20%
lanolin	15%
alcohol	3%
glycerin	3%
peanut or other vegetable oil	8%
mineral oil	2%
water to make up	100%

As you can see, the major ingredients of the mixture are oil and water. Glycerin and some of the other ingredients are added to prevent the oils from spoiling, and to extend the shelf life of the cosmetic. Some ingredients are also added to prevent the oil and water from separating. Colorants and perfumes can also be added.

Many different oils are used in cosmetics; sometimes they are quite exotic, like mink oil or turtle oil, and some are quite familiar, such as olive oil or peanut oil, or even corn oil. There is no evidence that one oil is better than any other in general. There are some oils that are better in specific cases, but only you can determine which work best for you.

To find out which oil seems best for your skin you'll have to buy small samples and test them. I bought about four bottles at a health food store: sesame oil, olive oil, apricot-kernel oil, and avocado oil. I found that apricot-kernel oil and avocado oil worked best for me. I know they work best because I used each oil for a week as a cleanser, as a lubricant, and as a night cream. My skin seemed calmer, smoother, and more even-toned after the apricot-kernel oil. I now look for apricot-kernel oil in the cosmetics I buy. Some friends have told me that olive oil works best for them, and they prefer either the oil alone, or products with the olive oil in some formulation. However, many vegetable oils, used above, will encourage acne, especially bumps and whiteheads. Adding a tablespoon or so of mineral oil to each cup of vegetable oil will prevent this.

The reason for using any oil or cream at all is to counteract the symptoms of dry skin. The applied oils are a substitute or a replacement for your own oils that might be insufficient to protect your skin against the elements. They do this by keeping your skin soft and pliable and they also prevent the evaporation of the moisture from your skin cells.

Some of the cost of any cream is perfume. Expensive fragrances add a great deal to the cost of any cosmetic; only you can decide what is most important to you. If you like the color, fragrance, or texture of a cream, that's fine—if you're not allergic to any of those additional ingredients. But be sure that the cream actually works best on your skin. Don't confuse color, texture, or fragrance with action. The best cream for your skin may be an ordinary ointment that is perfume-free. Think of how much you will save; perhaps even enough to buy some wonderful fragrance to use without the cream.

Petroleum Jelly and Mineral Oil versus Vegetable and Animal Oils

We've all read that many doctors believe petroleum jelly is as good a skin oil as any other. We've also heard that petroleum jelly is not good for the skin. There are advocates on both sides of the controversy. When I started giving skin-care lectures, my picture appeared in a magazine. Soon after that I received a letter from a large mineral oil company, asking that I withdraw a statement I had made that vegetable oil is better than mineral oil; enclosed in the letter was a duplicate of a report on the use of mineral oil on the legs of an elderly woman.

This made me quite anxious, and I started to collect information. Nutritionist and skin-care expert Gary Null writes, "Mineral oil is a mild, bland type of oil used as base material for many types of cosmetics. It is the last choice among the oils as it has a tendency to do away with the skin's own oil. Therefore products which use extensive amounts of mineral oil are not recommended for those with dry skin problems." Several other experts agree.

It is easiest to understand in this way: Petroleum jelly is to mineral oil as margarine is to corn oil. Petroleum jelly is a thick form of mineral oil; just as margarine is essentially a thickened form of corn oil. In the thick form Vaseline provides a barrier and a strong dense protective covering for the skin. In its thin form, mineral oil, like corn oil, is a soothing liquid.

The controversy about the use of mineral oil for the skin is so vexing because in some cases mineral oil is very good for the skin, and in some situations it isn't. If there is no other oil available, mineral oil fulfills the requirements of a lubricant. But as a main emollient, or used as the only skin oil, mineral oil may have some inadequacies.

The oil glands of human skin are concentrated on the face, the shoulders and back, and the pubic area. The glands of the face are very active in youth, and they provide a rich, protective covering to the skin that keeps it moist. But when these glands cease to be as active, the skin can't manufacture its own oily covering and needs a replacement. The problem in using mineral oil as this main covering is that mineral oil is a thinner oil than the natural oils which the human skin provides; the thinner oil has a tendency to dilute and wash away natural oils rather than lubricating or protecting. But on places such as the elbows, knees, legs, thighs, stomach, and perhaps even the arms where there are few or no oil glands, then as water—any water at all—to a thirsty person, the mineral oil does help. It smooths and soothes.

Mineral oil seems especially helpful and soothing on the skin of older people who find that the richer vegetable or animal oils are too thick and greasy. Rubbed on the arms, feet, and shins where there are few natural oil glands, mineral oil can prevent flakes and rough skin.

Mineral oil might also be useful in the treatment of very oily skin. If an oily skin was coated with mineral oil, that mineral oil which mixes easily with all other oils would help to "wash away" the thicker oil, and perhaps some blackheads and some pore-clogging cell debris as well. Mineral oil is good for situations where there is too much oil, and where there is too little oil.

You may ask, "What oils are suitable for most skins—those not excessively oily or those that are just a little dry, and not papery-dry?" Vegetable oils are preferred by many skin experts. Gary Null writes about oils in this way: "Animal fat oils most resemble the natural secretions of the human body. The oils most often used in formulations to protect and maintain the skin's moisture are lanolin, codfish oil, mink oil, and turtle oil." Null also thinks that vegetable oils are next best for the skin, and goes on to say that no one vegetable oil is really more effective than any other.

The problem with animal oils is that so many human beings are allergic to them. The oil of the sheep, lanolin, is perhaps closest to that of the human being, but many people are allergic to lanolin, and cannot use it or any product that contains lanolin. Very few people are allergic to vegetable oil, and because it has a pleasant texture, no smell, and seems so nice and clean, as well as being acceptable to most people, it can probably serve as a basic lubricant and protective. However, olive oil and avocado oil are known to clog pores, which can bring on acne, if the oil is not diluted with a small amount of mineral oil.

Three-Oil Lotion

This is a light lotion that can be used as a moisturizer all over your face and body. It contains no preservatives, so it should be stored in the refrigerator. If you use it often—and you should—you might want to keep some in a small jar near your sink, and the major portion in your refrigerator.

¼ cup lecithin (available in health food stores)
¼ cup water
¼ cup vegetable oil (apricot-kernel oil works well in this recipe)

2 tablespoons white coconut oil
1 teaspoon mineral oil

This is an all-purpose cream/lotion that should be smoothed and patted gently on the face, hands, and body. It encourages a smooth surface, and will help the skin retain moisture. It has none of the waxy feel of heavy creams, and it can be used under makeup and cosmetics. Add more water if you find it too greasy; add more oils if you find the cream disappears too soon.

Oily Ideas for Luxe Looks

For these little beauty tricks all you need is a small jar of your favorite vegetable oil.

Smooth blusher: Dab oil on your cheeks where you want to concentrate the color of your blusher. It will insure the powder of the blusher staying where you want it to stay. It also helps the blusher to "blush" for several hours, instead of fading away.

Smooth concealing: Using a small brush, paint the skin beneath your eyes with oil. It will make the concealer go on more easily, without pulling the skin.

Color matchups: If you want to use your lipstick as a cream blusher, dab a spot of oil on your cheeks and use the lipstick as a blusher.

Eyelasher: Coat your lashes with oil every night. They'll grow longer and stronger. (Be careful that no oil gets in your eyes.)

Upper-lip: Be sure that you coat this part of your face with oil before washing with a soap; you can ward off those tiny feather lines for years.

Brow flasher: Brush a small amount of oil (castor oil is best) on your brows with an old toothbrush or mascara brush.

Temple oils: Always cover the outer edges of your eyes with oil. It will soften the skin to make crow's-feet less noticeable.

Root touch-ups: Give your hair a color treatment, and prevent color buildup by painting your hair with oil. Start about a half-inch from the roots. You can use a cotton swab dipped in oil, or a pastry brush.

Steam-facial: Warm a bit of oil over a bowl of hot water. Clean your face carefully, so that it is free of every bit of grime or old makeup. Smooth the warm oil on your face. Cover your face with a warm towel. (You can first use a plastic sheet to avoid getting the towel oily, but remember to cut a nose hole.) Wash off the warm oil and notice the glow.

Leg-sheens: After shaving your legs, coat them with vegetable oil. An extra dab on the inside of the knees and chapped skin will vanish, even in the winter.

Scents: Create your own perfume by boiling rose petals in a cup of water. After they are boiled down, just add an equal amount of oil to make scented lotion for your body.

Foot-savers: Coat your feet with oil before you wrap them in a warm towel, and rest your feet on a warm hot-water bottle. They'll be ready for a pedicure in about 15 minutes.

Clean-coating: Cover your hands with oil before you start a big cleaning job. If it is a big job, coat hands with petroleum jelly after the oil. It will keep the oil on your skin, and double the protection.

Nails: Treat your nails after removing the old polish and before applying the new coat. Soak them in warm oil for 10 minutes. You can easily push cuticles down after this treatment.

Knees, heels, and elbows: Dull, ashy, scaly skin on the knees, elbows, or heels will disappear with just a few coatings of oil.

Ears: Dry skin around your ears is unattractive and ugly. Rub your lobes with oil, and dab oil wherever the skin looks dry.

Summer-glow: Cover your shoulders with a light oil on a summer day or evening. It will help preserve any tan you might have.

How to Make Your Creams "Work"

But if you want your skin creams and cosmetics to work most effectively, you have to prepare your skin properly so it will be affected by the cosmetics. This requires some planning. To get a cosmetic to work on the upper layer of the skin, the cosmetic must be watery. The keratinized flat cells on the upper layer are dehydrated, and can only be softened with water. To test this, place a piece of callused skin in a small jar of oil; it will remain hard and leathery. But if you place the bit of skin in water, it will not dissolve but will become softer and more flexible. A soft, flexible texture is your goal for the upper layer of your skin.

When you cover your skin with a thick oil (such as petroleum jelly), you can protect it from evaporation on the surface of the skin, but no new moisture will be added.

To get water on your skin to keep it soft and flexible you must spray or splash your face with water, and then cover that coating of water—before it evaporates—with oil. That trapped layer of water will gradually moisten the hard, horny, keratinized cells of the skin, making it soft and moist. The soft, moist skin allows your creams to be more effective and your cosmetics will seem to be absorbed better; their effects will also last longer. If you spray your face with water before applying a moisturizer and then again before makeup, the makeup will look fresh hours longer.

To help any cosmetic or unguent to be its most effective you have to get it below the horny layer to the next layer of the epidermis. You can do this by using sugabrasion (described in detail on page 00).

— Wash your face carefully, but do not dry it.
— Apply a thin coat of a mild vegetable oil, such as olive oil, mixed with a few drops of mineral oil.
— Using ½ teaspoon of granulated sugar, rub the surface of your skin gently. Concentrate on rough or chapped areas that seem flaky or dry.
— Wash away the sugar and as much oil as possible with very warm water.
— Stimulate the skin as much as possible by tapping the skin gently with the fingertips. Start at the neck and move upward. The skin will become slightly pink.

Your skin is now ready to receive whatever cream you use.

You've thinned the surface or horny layer, and you have also brought the skin's blood supply to the surface. The skin, thinned and moistened, and softened with warm water, is less of a barrier because it is thinner and more open, and the pores have been cleaned out.

It is important not to move the skin away from its subcutaneous tissue when it is warm and moist. Skin, like all protein tissue, can be weakened with excess heat.

How to Apply Creams

If you read directions on cosmetic booklets or talk to some cosmeticians, you'll notice they insist that the only way to apply oil, cream, foundation, moisturizer—anything that goes on the face—is to apply it in an upward motion. The theory is that upward and outward will "fight gravity" and prevent the skin from sagging. There seems to be little evidence to justify this belief. During the application of cosmetic creams or lotions you should avoid moving or forcing the skin away from its original position in any way. Moving the skin would weaken the collagen fibers. It doesn't really matter if you move the skin upward, or downward, or sideways; it is moving the skin that is damaging.

The progressive loss of muscle tone, sagging of the muscles, and the loss of a bouncy, firm fat pad under the skin is part of the aging process. It is hard to imagine that upward stroking would change the muscles. The best method for applying cosmetics is the "no-stroke method." That means that you apply the cream or oils as close to where it should be as possible without trying to spread it at all.

Cosmetic Creativity

You would be surprised how easy it is to create your own cosmetic creams. In fact, you can make all of your basic cosmetics and skin-care lotions from just a few staples. It's easy, inexpensive, and lets you custom-tailor your cosmetics to your skin. Here's all you need. Each item is available in drugstores.

alum
witch hazel
water
zinc oxide
aspirin
alcohol
borax
oils

Slight changes in the combinations or proportions of these ingredients will determine what sort of cosmetic you make. Any of these combinations can and should be mixed with water to achieve the consistency that you like best.

Always use glass or ceramic jars or bottles to mix your creams; shake or mix the ingredients well before each use. These cosmetics don't have any emulsifiers or stabilizers and the ingredients will separate. Make very small quantities, and store any extra in your refrigerator.

9

Hands and Hair

Hair Structure

Everyone wants strong, bouncy, shiny hair. Long hair, which grows from the scalp, can reach 4 or 5 feet in length. Short hair grows in the armpits, pubes, nostrils, and sometimes the ears. Brows and lashes are also examples of short hair. Lanugo hair—a soft, colorless down—grows all over the body and is almost invisible at times.

Hair is a wire-shaped structure composed of over 90 percent protein—the same kind of protein that is on the surface of the skin and constitutes your nails. The color of the hair varies with its chemical composition; light blond hair contains less carbon and hydrogen than brunette hair, but it contains more oxygen and sulfur.

Hair has two sections: the root, which is located beneath the surface of the skin, and the shaft, which is the part that we see. Hair grows at the rate of 6 inches a year. There are about 1000 hair follicles in every inch of your scalp, and you might have as many as 100,000 hairs on your head. If your hair is coarse, you may have fewer hairs on your head; if it is fine and full, you may have more. You can't create more hair by shaving, or cutting in any special way; a hair can only grow where there is a follicle. When a hair dies it is replaced by a new hair that grows from the same follicle.

— Long hair—the kind that is on the scalp—averages ½ inch of growth a month.
— Short hair does grow faster, and trimming the ends of your hair can encourage growth.

— A woman's hair grows faster than a man's hair. We naturally shed between 50 and 100 hairs a day.
— Eyebrow and eyelash hair shed every four or five months and are replaced by new hair growth.

The color of your hair depends on the pigment in your hair; white or gray hair is only the absence of pigment. The texture of your hair is determined by the shape and size of each hair. In cross-section,

straight hair is round

wavy hair is oval

curly hair is almost flat and ribbonlike

Hair, like skin, can actually absorb moisture. Once the outer covering of the hair is damaged or weakened, hair becomes even more porous. Chemicals with a high pH (alkalines) are often used to weaken the outer covering of the hair so that the hair will accept dyes more readily. This is why dyed or straightened hair becomes fragile and breaks easily. Normal hair is very strong and has amazing flexibility.

Scalp and Skin

The part of your skin that covers your head is not only the host to your hair but is also very important to your entire complexion. Many facial skin problems start in the scalp. The health of your hair and scalp cannot be separated from the health of your skin.

Located in the follicle of each hair are small oil-producing sebaceous glands. They secrete sebum which lubricates the hair just as the oil glands on the face secrete sebum to protect the skin of the face. These sebaceous glands are affected by changes in the endocrine system as well as in the blood circulation.

Because the skin on the face and the scalp is served by the same blood supply and shares many of the same characteristics, stimulating one helps to keep the other healthy. Each time you comb or brush your hair you have the opportunity to encourage your hair to grow—and to make your skin glow.

The purpose of a scalp treatment is to improve the condition of the scalp and to keep the hair from breaking or weakening. You can give yourself a scalp treatment, which can be an extra-special treat if you give yourself your favorite facial at the same time (see pages 196–205). Here is a technique taught by George Michaels, who runs an exclusive salon for women who want long, shiny, healthy hair:

Scalp-Savvy

— Release your hair from any pins or clips.
— Bend over at the waist and starting at the back of the neck, comb the hair toward the crown of the head. Use a widetoothed comb. When hair combs easily, switch to a natural bristle brush and start brushing from the ends of the hair outward.
— You should brush only a few inches of hair at one time—not try to take long strokes from scalp to end of hair. That has a tendency to break the ends of the hair that are dry or weak. Hold your hair as you brush it so that it isn't tugged at the scalp.

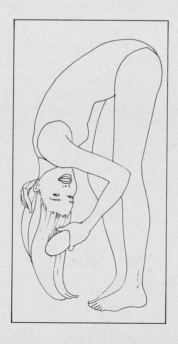

— Don't think you have to brush your hair those magic 100 strokes. Anywhere from 10 to 25 strokes, twice a day, is more than adequate. The idea of 100 strokes came from when hair was worn very long and every part of the hair had to be brushed with short, 6-inch strokes. Most women today do not have hair that is as long, nor as restrained, as when 100 strokes were popular.

— Stand up after combing and brushing. You'll notice that your face is flushed, and that it has been stimulated by the brushing.

The proper brushing of the hair will remove dust and dirt from the hair and give it added sheen; it will also loosen the dead surface skin of the scalp, dandruff. Leaning over when you brush or comb your hair has three purposes. It brings blood to the entire head, it makes the flow of blood to the face and head stronger, and it prevents the dead skin that is loosened by the brushing from falling on your face. Your skin is mostly protein, and when it dies, the dead protein is a wonderful diet for bacteria, and it collects old oil and dirt very easily. Don't let that dead skin accumulate on your scalp or fall on your facial skin.

The next step to stronger hair and smoother skin is to manipulate the scalp to loosen the scalp and under-muscles. Here are the steps:

1. Using a sliding motion, work your fingers up through your hair so they meet at the crown. Repeat two or three times.
2. Move the fingers up, but stop every few inches and pressing against the scalp, move slightly by rotating the skin.
3. Pay special attention to the front of the scalp and the hairline. Move the hair and scalp just at the hairline in short, circular motions. Repeat each motion once or twice, and then move on toward the crown.
4. Hold your hand on the side of your head, just above the ear and push against the hand. This is a form of isometric stress exercise that will work the muscles in the neck as well as the scalp.
5. Take a large handful of hair and gently tug it. Don't pull hard or jerk the hair. Just pull gently. It will strengthen and lengthen the hair.

If you do have a dandruff problem, remember it can come from either a too dry or too oily scalp condition. Both conditions are helped by frequent washing, and ridding the scalp of the excess scurf, as it is called.

Never wear anything tight on your hair or head. It will weaken your hair and sabotage any skin program you have. The pulling of a tight hairstyle, or the irritation of a tight hat, can constrict the free-flowing blood supply, giving you a headache and eventually, weak hair.

If you ever use a conditioner, or other scalp treatment that involves heat, or a warm moist towel, be sure that you spread a beauty mask on your face at the same time. You'll get an added bonus from the mask and the treatments to your face and scalp will amplify each other.

Shampoo

Everyone agrees that it's important to clean your hair correctly—it affects everything from your complexion to your mood. (Even the best professional makeup cannot compensate for dirty, oily hair.) I know a woman who dreads having a face-lift, not because of the discomfort of the surgery, nor because she fears the scars—only because she doesn't think she could stand going more than two days without a shampoo.

Hair-washing should be simple. Like face-washing, it is an early learned skill, and most people do it the same way—alas, the wrong way—for years. The most common mistake is too much shampoo or soap, and the next-most common mistake is not enough rinsing. And the wrong technique in shampooing can actually do more damage to your hair than cleaning your hair can benefit it. Here are some of the basics for a proper shampoo:

The Place   You'll want as much fresh water running through your hair as possible, so use a shower, or if that isn't convenient, get one of the shower-head attachments on a hose that can bring a spray of water directly to your hair. Don't wash your hair under a narrow, direct source of water; it can irritate your scalp and there is a tendency not to rinse evenly with a narrow water source.

The Water   Use the coolest water that is comfortable for you. Your hair strands weaken when they are wet, heat weakens them further. Always give your hair a final rinse of very cool water; it will hold its set longer. Besides—hot water doesn't clean any better than cool water. It is the shampoo that is cleaning your hair, not the water.

The Cleanser   The shampoo that you select must be adapted to your hair and your scalp condition. The condition of your scalp, and the color and treatments you've used on your hair, determine the product you should buy. Remember, it isn't the frequency of shampooing that can harm your hair—it is the way it is accomplished.

Check the product you've decided to use for alkaline/acid balance. It should have a pH of 4.0 to 5.5. If it is higher, you'll have to have an acid-neutralizing rinse, such as vinegar or lemon juice, to coat the hair and bring it back to its normal pH.

Before shampooing comb your hair carefully so that it is free of snarls, and brush the scalp to loosen any cells or other dirt or debris that might have gotten on your hair.

Pre-rinse your hair. Soak it completely for at least half a minute under the tepid water. The more thoroughly your hair is pre-rinsed, the less shampoo you'll have to use, and the cleaner your hair will be after just one washing. If you want, mix a little of the shampoo with some warm water, so it is less concentrated. Do not apply a glob of shampoo directly on the top of your hair—it will be very hard to distribute evenly.

Smooth the shampoo over your hair and start working it into the base of the hair growth, around the scalp. Rub quickly and firmly using only the cushions of your fingers. Work around your ears, temples, and the nape of the neck more than the crown of the scalp.

Dr. Jerome Litt, in his new book, *Your Skin & How to Live In It* (Ballantine Books, 1984), suggests that you treat your hair just as you would a fine sweater. He says, "How long would a sweater last if you were to constantly wash, comb, brush, color, tint, bleach, tease, twist and curl it?" He goes on to recommend very long leisurely shampoos of at least five minutes for oily hair. He believes that it is one of the most important and least stressed facts that to derive any benefit from a shampoo the agent must be massaged into the scalp.

Try to avoid tangling your hair during the lathering stage. Be very careful that you don't pull or tug at your hair; you might not feel or notice the damage until later.

Rinse

Always rinse again after you think you've rinsed enough. Remember how often you have to rinse your face, just to rid it of potential alkaline soap scum. Treat your hair the same way. After rinsing your hair should look and feel "squeaky" clean. Make your final rinse as cool as possible to close the outer covering of the hair strand.

Conditioner

Put on any conditioner just as you applied the shampoo. Work it in evenly, mixing it with water, if you need to, and gently squeezing it into the hair, working it from your hairline to the nape of your neck. Then, rinse the conditioner completely out of your hair. Be sure to rinse thoroughly.

Drying

Towel dry your hair by patting it and rolling it inside two layers of towels. If you can, avoid any blow-drying of your hair; or only blow-dry at the coolest setting for the finish. When your hair is wet it is greatly reduced in tensile strength and you can easily break your hair if you're not very careful. When the hair is more dry than damp, you can comb it gently, from bottom to top, in order to disentangle it more easily.

Styling

Don't brush your freshly cleaned hair. Comb it carefully, using a wide-toothed comb that is made of plastic, horn, ivory, or shell. Never use a metal comb on your hair, and check all of your combs for the smallest snag that might catch even one strand of hair.

You can clean your combs easily by adding a little baking soda to the wash water and then sloshing the combs through the mixture.

Hot Rollers

You should take as many precautions as possible when you use heat on your hair—especially hot rollers. Don't use hot rollers on dirty hair, and dampen your freshly cleaned hair before you apply the rollers.

After taking the rollers out, let your hair cool before you comb out the curls. The set will last longer, and the hair will be stronger. If you have a tendency to split ends, wrap the ends of your hair in paper before rolling around the heated curlers.

Philip Kingsley, a London-based trichologist (specialist in hair care) who has recently opened a branch of his salon in New York, works with such famous clients as Candice Bergen to create healthy hair for their busy life-styles. He uses a treatment that includes massaging a cream composed of olive oil, salicyclic acid, and other ingredients into the scalp. The salicylic acid rids the scalp of dandruff; the olive oil coats the strands of hair and helps to retain moisture. This cream is then set with moist heat. You can try an adaptation of this treatment in your own home, before your next shampoo. You will need:

½ cup olive oil, or cas-
tor oil
12 aspirins, crushed

teaspoon of mayon-
naise

Mix the three ingredients together and apply to the hair before shampooing, but after combing, and then wrap with a plastic sheet. Cover the plastic sheet with a warm towel. Allow to remain on the hair for about 20 minutes. The oil coats the hair, smoothing the shaft and preventing evaporation of natural moisture. The aspirin loosens skin cells from the surface of the scalp, and helps to rid the skin of old dead scalp skin. Wash the treatment away with warm, not hot, water. Shampoo as usual.

Kingsley also cautions not to wear warm hats indoors; I caution not to wear tight hatbands or sweatbands—ever.

Hair-Raising Face-Lifts

Several varieties of "Hollywood face-lifts" have been described in books and articles. The devices—either tape, or a series of clips and pins—are designed to pull up at the skin near the ear or temple, and so tighten the skin of the entire face. These devices do work, but they exact a high payment for the little help they provide. Pulling at the skin in any way weakens the underlying skin structure, and prevents the free circulation of life-giving blood to the skin. With that knowledge, here is a method of giving yourself a very fast lift (although, unfortunately, perhaps a headache), if you want to take 10 years off your appearance quickly.

— Lean over and comb your hair downward, loosening the hair over the tops of the ears.
— Take small sections of hair near the front of each ear, and braid them carefully.

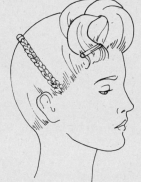

— Lift the two braids to the top of the head, pulling sharply on the braids so that they pull up on the surrounding skin.

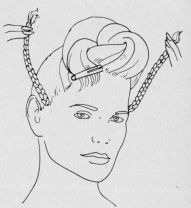

— Attach the braids to the top of the head and to each other with an elastic band to create tension.
— Comb some hair over the elastic band or cover the band with a decorative device, or hat.

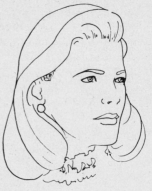

Do not use this technique often. It can weaken your hair, and it certainly will do very little for your disposition. It does work, however, and you might find the quick-lift so dramatic that you'll have to adjust your eye makeup, because the eye and brow area will be altered.

The Best Way to Part

Combing and brushing the hair are important steps in your personal grooming. The technique of arranging your hair is something that you have to master, because personnel department interviewers and employment agents notice a job candidate's hair before they notice anything else—even an impressive résumé! Clean, well-groomed hair is the single most involving feature you can have. What most people forget in arranging their hair is that the part—the basic division between sections of the hair—directs and controls the major design of the hairstyle. The following descriptions and illustrations can help you change the illusion of proportion and the contours of your face. It can minimize a less than perfect facial feature, it can make your hair look thicker, thinner, fuller, longer, or even show highlights and hair color more effectively.

To decide the correct position for the part of your hair, you have to take into consideration several factors. To do this, comb your hair smoothly away from your face over the top or crown of the head, and let it fall freely. Then shake your head and notice how the hair falls naturally. Are there any cowlicks, or irregular patterns, of growth? Notice where your hairline seems the most even, or where it might be thinning, or looking less than attractive. You'll have to work with your natural advantages, and draw attention away from imperfect features.

The most common ways to part the hair are:

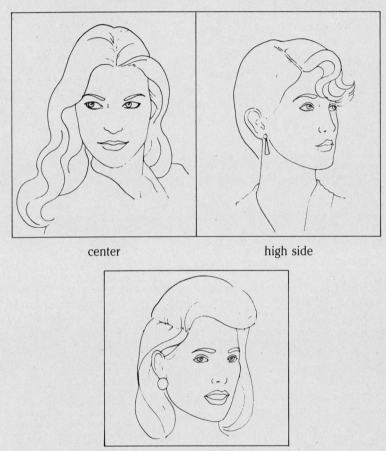

center   high side

low side

There certainly are other ways to part your hair, and you should experiment until you find one you like. It may be what your nose, chin, or forehead needs to make your face perfectly proportioned.

- Stress causes a weakening in the front hairline. If your forehead is receding, avoid any pulling clips or pins, and check with a doctor who is a specialist in the function of the endocrine gland. A curved rectangular part can create bangs to hide this flaw, however. If your forehead is narrow, cut deeply on the sides so that the bangs are long and wide. If face is wide, cut narrow bangs so that the sides of the face are hidden, narrowing the entire face. If your face is square, avoid square-cut bangs; have a little angle on them. And if your jaw is too wide, even it off with a wide fluffy bang on the top of your face; it will balance the dimensions.

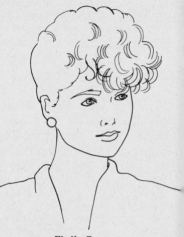

Fluffy Bangs

- To modify a wide or square face with a strong jawline, or an uneven hairline with weakening on one side, comb a diagonal part that runs across the top of the head, from one side of the forehead to the crown on the other side of the head. The diagonal part can be used to give a feeling of height to a round face, or to fill out a crown that is poorly shaped. It is also good for a square face, because anything as symmetrical diverts attention from a rectangular jaw.

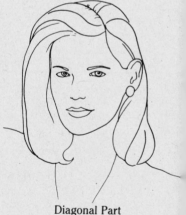

Diagonal Part

• To create height or width in any area of the scalp, simply part the hair, pin near the part, and double back the hair. This creates an arch of hair as an underpinning to height. It is a good alternative to the old-fashioned back-combing. A concealed part, used for height, is best with a one-sided style.

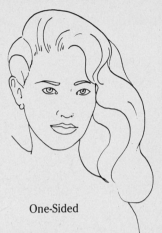

One-Sided

• Wispy hairs that fall from the hairline to the forehead can create an illusion without using too much hair. They are informal and young-looking. The wispy tendrils have to be as well-planned as a veil, to create a casual but neat effect. Brush the tendrils away from a center part if you have a heart-shaped face. For a narrow face, direct the wisps almost horizontally across the face; this works well for a narrow forehead, too. The square face should have uneven-length tendrils—avoid any sort of geometric effect.

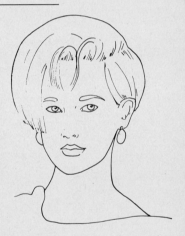

Wispy Bangs to Cover Forehead

Side parts, used for creating an illusion of height, should be near the middle of the forehead so that the eye is brought upward. To narrow the forehead, keep the width of the style well below the part.

Keep the fullness of your hairstyle near the narrowest part of the face, and flat hair to the widest part of your face.

Nice Nails

Nails are the keratin plates that grow on the ends of our fingers and toes. Like the skin's epidermis and the hair, they are composed mainly of protein cells; packed together they are whitish and translucent. This allows the color of the skin to show through the nail. Nails do not contain either nerves or blood vessels, but they can be an indication of general health.

Nail growth starts at the nail root, and a nail grows about ½ inch every four months. Like skin and hair, nails grow faster in warm weather. The nails on the hand you use most grow the fastest, and your third-finger nail grows faster than your thumb. Finger nails grow almost twice as fast as toe nails.

A good manicure can change the appearance of your hands, and should be the final touch in grooming. It should take no more than 15 to 20 minutes a week to keep your fingers and toes perfectly tended.

Brittle Nails That Split and Break

Nails, like hair and skin, need moisture and are protected by oils. On cold windy days when you're not wearing gloves your nails can become dehydrated and brittle—and then they split and layer easily. Nail polish remover is a powerful degreaser, and overuse of polish remover can also lead to splitting. But age and heredity are the real culprits.

Most nail problems come from infected cuticles because the cuticles have been cut incorrectly—or worse, picked and pulled. The cuticle is dead skin, but it is usually attached to live skin, and pulling at the cuticle tears the skin and leads to an infection.

Other nail problems come from allergic reactions to nail polishes and laquers. The nails themselves are not affected, but it is not infrequent to develop an allergic reaction from the wet nails if you touch your skin with them—just a touch of the tacky nail to your neck, face, or eyelid can lead to a rash.

Gelatin, minerals, and other nail-builders don't work well. If you want to strengthen your nails tap them, type, or play the piano. The slight jarring of the nails will actually strengthen them. It makes the nail bed defend itself, and the nails grow thicker. If you tap too much, your nail may thicken too much—just as age and too-short shoes sometimes bring on a thickening of your toe nails.

Hand Massage

Hand care should include a weekly hand massage to keep fingers soft and flexible. Care should be taken to keep the hands and nails moistened with oils and creams during the massage, or, as in facial massage, the skin's connective tissue can be weakened. Here are the steps:

1. Hold one hand in the other, carefully working the oil into each finger as well as the back of the hand.
2. Flip the hands back and forth to limber the wrists. Holding one finger at a time bend each finger at the joints slowly. Work from the tips toward the palm. Massage and gently bend the thumb as well.
3. Rest one elbow on a table or hold it firmly and massage the heel of the thumb. Gently draw the fingers, pulling them slightly and gently pinching the fingertips.

A massage with a light, warmed oil, followed by about 15 minutes inside of a plastic wrap or bag, will ready your hands and nails for a perfect manicure. An added benefit is that massaging the hands during cold winter months seems to increase the blood supply, and helps your fingertips resist the coldest weather.

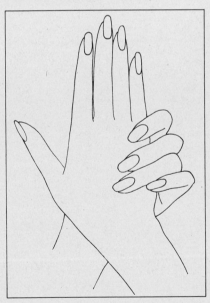

Hand Care

The word *manicure* comes from the Latin word for hands, *mani*. A manicure should improve the appearance of the skin and nails and keep the hands youthful and smooth. Hand care is easy and practical at home. You will need this equipment:

> Soft wooden sticks called orangewood sticks
> Nail file
> Small scissors
> Clippers
> Emery boards
> Nail buffer (optional)
> Nail brush (optional)

You'll also need these basic supplies:

> Oil (vegetable oil is as good as hand lotion)
> Soap or cleansers
> Nail polish remover
> Pumice stone
> Nail-polish thinner
> Base coat polish
> Liquid nail lacquer
> Saucer or shallow bowl
> Cotton
> Toothpicks
> Tissues

Basic Home Manicure

Before starting your manicure, wash your hands carefully, clean the nails with a brush, and then massage the hands with warm oil.

1. Starting with the little finger of the strong hand, remove any old polish. You can do this with a tiny wad of cotton soaked in polish remover and pressed over the nail to the count of 10 to soften the polish. Wipe the cotton from the cuticle to the tip of the nail. Try not to smear the softened polish into the corners of the nail or into the cuticles.

2. When the nails are free of polish, shape them with a file and the emery board. Make the general shape of the nail conform to the shape of the finger and fingertip.

- An oval almond-shaped nail for most hands.
- A slender hand requires tapering longer nails.
- A strong broad hand is best balanced by a square or rectangular nail with only the corners slightly rounded.
- A round or broad nail should be encouraged to grow as much as possible by gently smoothing the edges.

3. Soften the cuticles after filing by immersing the fingers, one at a time, in a mixture of warm soapy water. Dry the fingers and push back the cuticles, one finger at a time. Use the orange-wood stick to avoid scratching the softened nail. Also, avoid excess pressure on the nail base.

4. Use a bit of cotton wound around a toothpick, moistened with warm soapy water, to clean the underside of each nail. If you leave the nails unpainted, you can whiten this overhanging edge with a solution of hydrogen peroxide, or with one of the cream bleaching preparations.

5. Rinse away all oil and soapy water from the fingers with a clear, cool rinse of fresh water. Then steady the hand on a table and examine the nails to be sure they are the shape and length you want.

6. Starting with the little finger, apply a base coat of polish to each nail, working from cuticle to tip in a smooth stroke. Allow the base coat to dry until it can be touched without smudging.

7. Apply the nail enamel after dipping the brush into the polish and wiping off any excess on the edge of the bottle. Cover the nail evenly in rapid, smooth, sweeping strokes from the base to the nail tip.

8. Remove any excess polish from the sides of the fingers with a toothpick wrapped in cotton and dipped in polish remover. Apply a sealer coat over the polish, and stroke around and under the tips of the nails for added support and protection.

9. Allow the nails to dry thoroughly. (Dip hands in cold water to harden nails rapidly.) Coat the hands and fingertips with hand lotion.

Nail Repairs

There are some basic repairs that you can perform to save some nail "disasters," and preserve your manicure.

To Restore a Broken Nail (keep broken tips in a clean glass jar)

1. Place a thin, flat wisp of tissue paper, soaked in mending fluid, (many professional manicurists use Crazy Glue) on the nail. It should extend over the edges slightly.
2. Place the broken nail tip (from that nail, or from some other) over the cotton.
3. Dip a toothpick in liquid remover and use it to turn ends of tissue or cotton back over the nail tip. This will cover the edges of the break.
4. Saturate another strip of tissue with mending fluid and apply across the nail to anchor the tip, and tuck in under the nail. Smooth the surface.
5. After the fluid dries thoroughly, file bumps gently, coat with a base coat, and then polish.

To Repair a Split Nail

1. You can use a small piece of special mending tissue, or a piece of tissue paper soaked in mending fluid. Place it horizontally over the split in the nail.
2. Tuck the tissue under the nail, using a toothpick, and smooth the patch (away from the nail edge) with the toothpick.
3. Dry the patch completely before applying the base coat and a new coat of polish.

Nail News

- If you have poor circulation, and cold fingers and toes, try buffing your fingernails and toenails. It increases the circulation of the blood to the fingertips.
- To make wide nails appear longer and narrower, apply the lacquer only to the center of the nail.
- Bleach stains from fingertips with cream bleach that is used for

facial hair. Simply paint on stained spots, leave on for about 5 minutes, and then wash away.

- Always allow a tiny margin of cuticle to remain at the base of your fingers. It will prevent a fringe of loose skin from forming a pocket.
- You can use a pumice stone lightly on ridged nails to smooth them before buffing or polishing. Wet the pumice stone slightly to avoid damaging the nail.
- White spots on a nail do not indicate disease. They are caused by injuries to the base of the nail. As the nail continues to grow they will disappear.
- Many women report their nails and hair seem to grow faster when they diet. (It may be because dieters usually try to get more protein in their diets.)
- Nail lacquers or polish removers contain solvents that have a very drying effect on the nails, and strip the natural oils in the nails. To offset the drying action of the remover, soak fingers in warm oil right after removing polish.

Pedicure

Before you put on those new sandals be sure your feet are ready to "walk in beauty." Besides making you look better, a pedicure can make a real difference in how you walk and how you feel.

Equipment

You'll need the same tools for a pedicure as for a manicure, plus a few extras.

1. Comfortable place where you can put your feet up
2. Files
3. Oil (for massage)
4. Toenail nippers, scissors, files
5. Cotton and tissues

Preparation

1. Remove old polish from the toenails.
2. Clip and file the nails. Shape the nails straight across; don't cut or file the corners. Smooth the rough edges with fine emery board.
3. Using a pumice stone or specially prepared callus or foot-file, pare down rough spots, corns, and calluses.
4. Soak your feet in warm soapy water and brush the soles gently.
5. Remove feet and pat dry. Using an orangewood stick, loosen the cuticles around each toe. Cover each foot with a layer of warm oil.
6. Massage each foot, starting at the instep and working toward the toes. Hold the foot in your hands, rotating the skin with your thumbs. After loosening the feet, pull gently on each toe. Relax and rotate feet at ankles.

To Polish

1. Weave tissue between your toes to separate them, or insert cotton or tissues between toes. Remove any oil from your toenails by wiping them with nail-polish remover.
2. Apply polish and allow polish to dry. If you're in a hurry, polish will set very quickly if you can chill the polish in the refrigerator before using to thicken it slightly.
3. After polish is dry, coat your feet and ankles with "Three-Oil Cream" (see page 170).

10

Easy, Fast, and Effective Do-It-Yourself Cosmetics

For several years I've been collecting formulas and recipes for home-made cosmetics. I've found that many of them work remarkably well, but too many of the recipes require exotic ingredients and complicated preparations. The formulas I've included here are all easy and fast to clean up after. They are usually based on applying an oil, an astringent (a slight irritant), or an abrasive to the skin. When you use any of these recipes, mix in some caution; just as you can be allergic to commercial ingredients, you can also suffer an unwanted reaction from the use of foods or produce as cosmetics.

Mix very small quantities in a glass or in a ceramic cup, and don't at-tempt to store kitchen cosmetics in your refrigerator for more than a day. The foods will deteriorate.

Some of the concoctions are messy to apply. Commercial cosmetics are formulated to have just the right consistency, color, and smell—in using food products you have to forgo that convenience. On the "up side," food cosmetics sometimes bring a more dramatic improvement because they're not diluted, and you can probably avoid unwanted side effects because there are so few ingredients.

I hope you enjoy the recipes—and profit from the results.

Skin-Care Menu

BASIC CITRUS CLEANSER

(For Oily Skin)
(about 6 weeks worth—
this stores well in the refrigerator)

1 tablespoon grapefruit juice	6 tablespoons petro-leum jelly
¼ teaspoon borax	

Over a very low flame heat the grapefruit juice. Mix in the borax. In a small egg poacher melt the petroleum jelly until liquid. Mix the citrus and borax combination and the liquid petroleum jelly together and beat well. Transfer to a shallow jar. Use instead of soap on cold winter days. Remove with rinses of very warm water.

KEYBOARD CLEANSER

(Especially Good for Hands)

2 tablespoons glycerin	2 tablespoons water
2 large lemons, squeezed for juice	2 drops hydrogen of peroxide

Mix together in a pretty bottle, and shake well before using. Use carefully on the hands and face, for bleaching of discolored skin.

ALMOND BLISS

(A Cooling Skin Refresher)

¼ pound shelled almonds	2 cupfuls clean, soft water

Chop the almonds and mix thoroughly with the water. Boil together for about 10 minutes until a milk is formed. Bottle, and store in cool place.

MAGIC ALMOND MASK
(Not for Dry Skin)

6 egg whites (Use the sulfur-rich yolks for an oily-skin mask.)

½ pound pulverized almonds

The juice of 3 medium lemons

Mix all the ingredients together in a glass or ceramic bowl. This makes enough mask for about 4 treatments. Store in the refrigerator.

BREWER'S MASK
(For Oily Skin)

2 packets powdered yeast

2 tablespoons beer

Mix the yeast and beer together to form a mask. Apply to skin for no more than 10 minutes. Rinse off with warm water.

BUTTERMILK SKY
(To Tighten Sagging, Oily Skin)

¼ cup dry oatmeal
1 tablespoon yogurt

1 tablespoon milk

Mix together and apply to your skin. Leave on about 10 minutes. (If it gets messy, apply a damp handkerchief over the mask to keep the mask moist and to control it.) Rinse off with warm water.

EXECUTIVE CLEANSER
(This Is Great for Stress-Dried Skin)

¼ cup apricot-kernel oil

3 drops cologne

Mix together, and apply to face. The cologne is just to make the oil smell nice. After applying, place a plastic sheet with a nose hole for breathing over the oily face. Relax for 10 minutes. Wash away.

FAST-TRACK PICKUP

½ ripe avocado

Slice the avocado into very thin slices. Lie down and place the slices on the face. Place the slices directly over any tense or wrinkled areas. Relax for about 10 minutes. Throw the avocado slices away and rinse the face.

JOGGER'S OVERCOAT

(For Cold Weather)

1 tablespoon olive oil   petroleum jelly

Splash water on your face, or mist it with a spray. Cover the water with a coat of olive oil. Cover the olive oil with a thin coat of petroleum jelly. This layered protection will keep the moisture trapped on your skin. Wash off carefully and follow with an astringent to clean pores completely.

ONE IN ONE

(Skin Freshener)

1 tablespoon orange   1 tablespoon cooking
  juice   oil
1 teaspoon mineral oil

Mix together and pat on face. The slightly acid juice will freshen the skin. The oil prevents irritation.

ACNE IMPACT

(For Adult and Stress-Related Acne)

1 ounce powdered   1 pint rose water
  alum
1 tablespoon lemon
  juice, or 2 table-
  spoons apple cider
  vinegar

Mix together in small bottle. Shake before using. To use, saturate a cotton ball with the lotion, and swab the areas that are bumpy or have enlarged pores. This lotion can be used on nose, back, and other very oily areas.

COMPU CLEANSER

1 tablespoon Pepto-Bismol (an antacid)

Spread the liquid on the face. The product is slightly alkaline and will have a slight peeling effect.

BANANA BOOSTER

1 large banana

Cut the banana in half. Skin it and mash the fruit of one of the halves in a small bowl. Apply the fruit to the face, but avoid the eyes and mouth. Relax and eat the other half of the banana with a glass of warm water. (Sounds odd, but you'll feel quite good and look good after this booster.)

SWEET FACE

1 tablespoon honey   1 teaspoon milk for dry
1 teaspoon lemon for   skin
  oily skin

Mix the honey with either lemon or milk. Spread on face. Allow it to remain for 10 to 15 minutes. Rinse off with cool water.

AEROBIC ALERT

(Skin Toner and Freshener)

3 tablespoons almond   ¼ teaspoon alum
  extract
1 tablespoon white
  wine

Using a damp sponge, stroke the mixture over the face. Store in a small bottle in the refrigerator.

MILK-MADE

1 tablespoon yogurt   1 tablespoon powdered
                             milk

Apply to your skin and leave on about 15 minutes. If you can, cover with milk-dampened handkerchief to keep the mask moist. Rinse with cool water.

OVER TIME
(An Overnight Treatment)

¼ cup olive oil   ¼ cup avocado oil
¼ cup castor oil   1 teaspoon mineral oil

Mix the oils together. Slather the oils on the face, neck, hands, and arms. Wrap the arms in plastic wrap, put the hands in plastic bags, wrap the neck in plastic wrap, and relax for 15 minutes. Rub the entire body with a rough terry towel (you'll have to wash it afterward), and spray with cool water. Do not wash off.

GRAPE-NUTS GLOW

1 tablespoon Grape-   2 tablespoons butter-
   Nuts cereal   milk

Mix together and rub gently on your face and neck. It is a morning wake-up that will make you glow.

STIMU-SALAD

3 outer leaves of lettuce   3 very thin slices to-
   (the dark leaves are   mato
   best)
1 tablespoon mayon-
   naise

Spread the mayonnaise on the lettuce and place a slice of tomato on each leaf. Relax and place the combination tomato-side-down on your face. The lettuce will keep the tomato moist and active.

CALL ME IN THE MORNING

2 aspirins crushed be-
tween pieces of pa-
per

1 teaspoon face cream
or Crisco

Mix aspirins and cream together in the bowl of a spoon. Gently rub the slightly gritty substance across the nose, or other oily sections of the face. Avoid the eye area; do not use on throat. Wash off, and apply makeup.

BATHER-ER-CISE

(For Dry Skin)

½ cup sesame oil or
olive oil

2 capfuls detergent
shampoo

Pour a small amount under the faucet for each bath. Store in a cool, dark place.

FOOT FLARE

½ inch ribbon of toothpaste per foot

Rub toothpaste around your toenails and on the soles of the feet. Rinse with cool water.

PINEAPPLE SPLASH

½ cup fresh pineapple
juice (add crushed
pulp if you can)

½ cup milk

Fill a basin with water, add the mixture to the basin, and splash face with the pineapple-milk water. It will make skin tight and clean-feeling. It is drying, however, and must be followed by a moisturizer.

APPLE III

1 medium-sized apple   1 small handkerchief

Peel the apple and discard the peel. Grate or finely chop the apple. Place the apple inside the handkerchief. Press and squeeze against the skin. It will cleanse the skin and dissolve dead matter and old cosmetics. Rinse with cool water.

WHEAT WHIZ

¼ cup wheat germ   2 tablespoons olive oil
1 tablespoon sesame
  seeds

Crush the wheat germ and the sesame seeds together. Add the olive oil. Spread on the face. To keep the mask from drying out, cover the face with a moist gauze. Relax for about 15 minutes. Rinse the mask away with cool water. (This is only for dry skin. Both wheat germ and olive oil have been found to trigger acne.)

EGG SHAMPOO CONDITIONER
(For Skin and Hair)

2 eggs   1 ounce (a jigger) of gin
1 teaspoon olive oil

Mix the eggs, oil, and gin together. Apply to the ends of the hair, and wrap the hair in a warm, moist towel. Paint the solution on the skin and cover with a warm, damp face towel. Allow to remain for about 10 minutes. Wash away with cool water.

POTATO PACK

½ cup dehydrated pota-   Enough water to make
  toes   a paste
1 tablespoon glycerin

Mix together and apply to the face. It is a soothing, protective mask that is excellent for sensitive skin—dry or oily. Wash off with tepid water.

POTATO EYES

½ medium potato   cheesecloth or a thin
                                   handkerchief

Grate the raw potato into the handkerchief. Apply to the skin around
the eyes by forming it into a compress. A slice of raw potato can do the
same thing. You may find that scooping out a small depression in the
slice helps it stay on your eye. Place the depression on your eyeball
—it keeps the potato slice from slipping toward your ear.

80-PROOF RECIPES

RUSSIAN BREEZE
(For Blemished Skin)

1 cup water   1 teaspoon lemon juice
1 jigger vodka

Splash or spray mixture on face. Blot excess but don't wipe it off.

WINE TINGLE

1 tablespoon white   1 tablespoon red wine
   wine for oily skin   for dry or tired skin

Dip a cotton ball into the wine and dab on face. Allow wine to dry on
your face. Rinse away after about 15 minutes.

SLOW SKIN FIZZ

1 tablespoon cham-   ¼ teaspoon boric acid
   pagne
4 tablespoons witch
   hazel

Mix in a small bottle to use as a toner or freshener with cotton balls.

BRANDY BRACER

1 tablespoon brandy
(any kind)
3 tablespoons grape-
fruit juice

3 tablespoons water
1 tablespoon camphor
water

Mix together and apply with cotton or a sponge. For oily skin only.

MINTY JULEP
(Toner)

1 tablespoon crème de
menthe

2 tablespoons vegeta-
ble oil

Mix the alcohol and oil and tap gently into the skin.

STRAWBERRY TONIC

¼ cup strawberry pulp
1 jigger gin

1 teaspoon glycerin

Mix together and use as a tightening mask. Apply to face and let it remain for about 15 minutes. Rinse with warm water.

Peanut Better

Peanuts are one of nature's wonders. They are high in nutrient value and high in oils, but also often an acne-stimulator. Peanuts are 30 to 50 percent oil, and a pound of peanuts contains more protein than a pound of sirloin steak. Like all legumes, they play a key role in the assimilation of nitrogen from the air, and they can renew the earth when they are plowed under and used for fertilizer.

CREAM MASK

(To Moisturize)

1 tablespoon creamy-   1 teaspoon mineral oil
  style peanut butter

Mix the peanut butter with the mineral oil. Apply to the face. You can even apply this rich mixture to the eye area if you wish. Also apply it to the backs of your hands for super softening. Allow it to remain on the face for about 10 minutes. Wash away with very warm water.

CRUNCH RUB

(To Smooth and Soften)

1 tablespoon crunchy-style peanut butter

Apply the peanut butter to the skin and rub it gently over any rough spots. The peanut butter oils prevent the chunky nutmeats from being too rough, whereas the nutmeats act as an abrasive. Wash with very warm water.

Salty Skin

Salt attracts water. There are many other minerals or substances that attract moisture, but salt can easily be used with oil to make an excellent moisturizer. Use Dead Sea salt (available at health food stores) if possible, or any sea salt with this recipe:

Mix together ¼ cup vegetable oil and ¼ cup water and shake well. Apply to a damp face. After you apply the oil/water lotion, sprinkle salt on your face, or just on the area that you plan to moisturize. Don't rub the salt in—simply allow it to rest on the face for about 10 minutes. Rinse with warm water, and if the face seems too slick, use a light soaping, followed by repeated rinsing.

CZARINA'S SALT BATH

Every spring, before going to the Black Sea resorts, the Russian royalty used this formula to soften their skin. You'll need a damp linen or cotton dish towel, and a cup of salt. Dampen the towel in warm water, and dip the damp towel into the salt so some salt adheres to the towel. Stand in your tub, and working upward from the feet, gently rub the towel with the gritty salt over your body. Don't rub too hard; it should just make your skin feel tingly, not raw. After this treatment, cover your body with a vegetable oil, such as olive oil, and then rinse with very warm water.

MINERAL BATH

1 cup sea salt	1 cup epsom salts
1 cup baking soda	1 cup strong tea

Fill your tub about half full of warm water and then add this mixture, one cup at a time, stirring well. Get into your bath and lie back for about 5 minutes. Immerse your body as completely as you can. Add more water if needed. Stand and shower off the salts and then cover your body with coconut oil, a light vegetable oil, or mineral oil. Don't dry off before applying the oil.

JELLY MASK

It evens color, softens skin, smooths, hydrates, and pulls off dead skin cells. This mask will keep for several weeks without refrigeration, and it is best if you buy all the ingredients at the health food store. Use a double boiler, or set a small glass jar in boiling hot water to keep the mask ingredients warm and liquid while you are mixing, but do not boil. It takes about 5 minutes to make this mask, and it is more potent than any commercial cosmetic mask available.

½ cup strong herbal tea   ¾ cup dry pectin
(See p. 166–169 for a list
of herbs and a description of how they can be
used for your own complexion needs.)
½ cup powdered glycerin

Place the glycerin in a glass jar. Place the jar in the boiling hot water, and wait until the glycerin liquifies. Add the pectin very slowly, and blend with a wooden or glass mixer until the powder dissolves. Add the hot tea very slowly, a little at a time, and mix carefully after each addition. Keep the mixture in a double-boiler until all the ingredients are well combined. Pour into warm jars and allow to cool overnight or at least several hours before using.

To use this mask, paint it on with a small pastry brush or a large, soft paintbrush (always wash the brush right after using it). Allow the mask to harden for about 15 minutes, and then remove with alternating rinses of warm and cool water. If the jelly is applied thickly enough, the mask can often be peeled off. When you peel it off, be careful not to pull delicate skin with the mask. This mask will pull off dead cells and will clear your pores, but it is not drying or harsh. Do not use near the eyes; peeling the mask off might be too violent for the thin skin.

"Natural" Cosmetics

No cosmetics are really natural. Any processing to preserve a product makes it "unnatural" and often better. But, there are some ingredients that you can and should use directly from nature, which will give you fast cures for some very annoying skin problems.

Fruits and vegetables are part of every healthy diet. Various vegetables and fruits naturally include chemicals that are beneficial to human skin. The chart below includes only a few of the fruits, plants, and herbs that are useful in treating your skin. It is important to do as little as possible to these vegetable substances; the soothing, calming, and healing elements can be destroyed by heating too much or mixing them too vigorously. The only exceptions are dried herbs, which should be steeped in boiling water to release their beautifying potential.

Young, Oily, Blemish-Prone Skin

Apple
What it does: Brightens, clears and firms. Slightly astringent. Do not use on the eye area or under the nose.
Why: Phosphorus, calcium, iron, potassium.

Blackberry
What it does: Astringent, will make your skin feel tight and soothed when crushed and applied to the skin. The juice will stain. If you eat blackberries in quantity, they can be a mild diuretic and rid your body of excess water.
Why: Tannin, iron, some acids.

Grapefruit
What it does: Temporarily tightens large pores. Dab a bit on the nose and see your pores seem to vanish; excellent as a diluted wash for blotchy complexions. Add a

Grapefruit (cont'd)	bit to your rinse water when washing your face, either juice, or just a few crushed sections. *Why:* Citric acid to keep the skin bacteria-free, natural sugars for healing.
Iris	*What it does:* Soothes and calms skin; if you have any plants, take some of the blossom petals and place them on your face; cover with a warm, moist cloth. *Why:* Leaves and petals contain tannin.
Lemon ✓	*What it does:* Bleaches discolored skin, tightens large pores, helps skin maintain its mantle. Do not use without diluting with water; too acidic to be used directly. *Why:* Citric acid, sugars, and vitamin C for cell health.
Mint	*What it does:* Crush leaves with mortar and pestle; place between layers of gauze, and moisten with water. Use as a natural mask for smooth, poreless skin. *Why:* Menthol in its natural form tightens the pores; mint has its own natural oils and a good supply of iron.
Strawberry	*What it does:* Blemished skin can be cleaned and cleared with a crushed strawberry mask. Teeth and gums are invigorated by rubbing with the pulp of the berry. *Why:* Salicylic acid is one of the components of strawberries, which rids the skin of dead cells; iron, lime, and sodium are also in the berries.
Pineapple	*What it does:* Cleanses and freshens skin; a strong toner. Mix the juice with washing water, or rinse water. Rub the fruit on feet for a clean and tingling sensation, and to rid the feet of dead skin and calluses. *Why:* Contains protein-digesting enzyme; also is anti-inflammatory.
Tomato	*What it does:* Helps to dislodge blackheads and cleans blocked pores. Use a slice of tomato over irritated areas to soothe puffy or irritated skin. *Why:* Acidic, it restores natural balance of the skin.
Yeast	*What it does:* Enlivens sallow, dull skin; keeps pores clear of sebum plugs and makes skin look glowing and firm. Stimulates regeneration in cells. *Why:* High in vitamin B complex, it also contains phosphorus, potassium, protein, and lipids—the fats that are important to all cell function.

Dry, Rough, Aging Skin

Almond

What it does: The oil is perfect for dry skins; even the ground nut meat can be used on the most delicate skin as a nondestructive abrasive. The husks are also perfect abrasives.
Why: The almond meat is a lubricant with useful oils; contains vitamin A and calcium.

Artichoke ✓

What it does: Invigorates skin that needs oxygen, bleaches pigmented areas and spots; eating it helps rid the body of fat deposits; cleans the blood.
Why: Contains mineral salts, proteins, vitamin B; high content of iodine (can stimulate an outbreak of acne).

Birch

What it does: Collect birch bark, sliver it up, and boil it into a tea; use in baths or in washing. Birch will calm rashes, and soothe any kind of chapping or allergic reaction.
Why: Contains sodium, resins, tannin, phosphorus. Was used by American Indians for all kinds of skin problems.

Cabbage

What it does: Holds moisture in skin when leaves are used over a mask. Cabbage has slight disinfectant quality.
Why: Contains sulfur, iodine, vitamins A and D. This is a humble but potent vegetable.

Carrot

What it does: A poultice of grated or shaved carrot will hydrate the skin and will clean and clear away dead skin cells. If you use a bit of mayonnaise, the carrot will adhere to the skin. Carrot is an excellent moisturizer, and carrot juice can be mixed with an oil for an enriching mask.
Why: Contains vitamin A, iron, iodine, potassium, lime.

Fennel ✓

What it does: Calms and soothes discolored skin; leaves an even-toned complexion in place of blotchy skin. Mix fennel in your favorite commercial mask, or make a fennel and oil mask. It will soothe too-high color, and as a vascular constrictor it will help broken veins.
Why: Iron, phosphorus, and lime are just three of the minerals in this herb.

Grapes	*What it does:* Slightly diuretic, they have a regenerating and healing effect on the skin; they can help heal bruised or chapped skin. *Why:* Contains sugars, vitamins A, B, and E.
Potato	*What it does:* A nutrient and mild tonic for skin, it can help rid the skin of retained water and bags under the eyes. *Why:* Potassium, starch, vitamin C.
Seaweed	*What it does:* Wonderful for dehydrated skins, it reduces fat accumulation where you don't want it (under the chin, for example) and firms the skin. If you're at the ocean, take some seaweed home and let it float in your bath. Wrap it on the face or arms, and you'll notice the skin tighten and firm. High in iodine, avoid seaweed if you have a tendency to acne. *Why:* Protein, oils, a mucilage coating, and iodine are all in seaweed.
Wheat	*What it does:* Stimulates dehydrated, rough skin; use wheat in any mask and add to your own creams. Wheat is a calmer for sensitive skins, and reduces inflammation. Beware: wheat can stimulate an allergic reaction. *Why:* Wheat contains proteins, iron, albumin, and potassium.
Rhubarb	*What it does:* Juice from raw rhubarb can brighten and tone faded skin and tighten large pores. (Don't eat any of the leaves; the stalks can be eaten, but the leaves are toxic.) *Why:* Contains malic acid, which is strongly acidic and almost peels the dead skin away; also contains some natural sugars as well as a natural bleach, which can be irritating if left on the skin.

Sensitive, Temperamental, Delicate Skin

Apricot	*What it does:* The powdered pit (seed) can be rubbed against the skin to soothe and rid the skin of dead cells. Pulp is a good moisture mask for all skin types. *Why:* Rich in vitamin A.

Blueberries	Excellent for very sensitive skin, the berries relieve congestion and a poultice of crushed berries can even be used in the eye area. Astringent and anti-inflammatory action. (Stains clothing and skin.) *Why:* Natural menthols and tannin; there is also salicylate, which speeds the emergence of new cells.
Chamomile	*What it does:* A tradition in France for relieving inflamed skin; helps stop dehydration, relieves sunburn, and is a slight bleach. Use chamomile tea bags to reduce puffy eyes. *Why:* Lime, potassium, and azulene (a blue hydrocarbon) that comes from the chamomile blossoms.
Cucumber	*What it does:* This slightly astringent vegetable works wonders when applied around the eyes. For a real cellulite fighter, spread cucumber slices on upper thighs, buttocks, or hips and wrap in plastic wrap for 15 minutes. *Why:* Mildly astringent; acts as diuretic when eaten in quantity.
Eggplant	*What it does:* Soak some slices of eggplant in water; apply to skin for a moisturizing mask. Helps to fight dehydration. *Why:* High in vitamins A and C.
Marigold	*What it does:* A real boon to blotchy skins, it can be used for burns and sunburns as well as eczema and rashes. Pound the leaves into a pulp and apply to face; marigold has an antiseptic effect. *Why:* Antiseptic and encourages healing without scar formation; contains salicylic acid, mucilage, and sulfur.
Pear	*What it does:* Select a ripe pear and slice it into thin slices. Apply slices to inflamed or blotchy skin; it will calm almost immediately. A purifier and a soothing emollient. *Why:* Contains tannin and sugars.
Rose	*What it does:* Soothing and relaxing, especially for the eyes. Use rose petals over the eyes and cover with a damp cloth. This is especially good for dark circles under eyes. Rose petals are both astringent and a tonic to the skin. *Why:* Contains essential oils and tannin.

Soybean
cakes (tofu)

What it does: Very moisturizing for dry, dehydrated skin. The soybean has a high percentage of oil, and is especially important to very dry, papery skin. Good on throat, eyes, and mouth areas.

Why: Contains proteins, oils, lecithin, amino acids, nitrogen, vitamins A, B, E.

Turnip

What it does: Dry, rough, and blotchy skin as well as rosy, inflamed skin can be helped by a compress of grated turnip. It is a vasoconstrictor, which means that it acts to tighten the skin's capillaries. It also helps in healing and reduces scar tissue.

Why: Contains vitamins B and C as well as sulfur and minerals. This is a standby in winter skin care.

Wheat germ

What it does: Thin, sensitive, dry skin and aging skin are helped by this almost immediately. Mix yogurt and some wheat germ, apply to face and neck, cover with a damp cloth, and relax. You will see a big change in about 10 minutes.

Why: Contains vitamin B and proteins. (Some people are allergic to wheat germ so be sure you test your reaction on a small patch of skin before covering your entire face.)

11

A Skin-Care Glossary

The more you know about any product, the more able you are to evaluate how well that product satisfies your needs and fulfills your expectations. Many of the terms used in this book are familiar in a very general way, but there are often misconceptions about the products and the ingredients used in most cosmetics.

This small glossary is designed to help clarify all the terms that are used, and to provide you with a resource for checking the labels of your own cosmetics or foods.

Most cosmetics include preservatives. These are necessary for protection against infection from bacteria, fungi, and yeast that might be attracted to the oils or organic substances such as lanolin in cosmetics.

The degree of acidity or alkalinity of a product is also important. Too acid, or too alkaline for your skin, and a cosmetic can cause irritation. Citric acid, from lemon juice or from apple cider vinegar, is very popular in homemade cosmetics just because it neutralizes the alkaline properties of cleansers or other products. Buffers such as calcium carbonate (chalk) are often added to cosmetics, also. The trick in selecting either commercially manufactured cosmetics or in making your own at home is finding the exact formula that will be most compatible with your own pH-acid-alkaline balance.

Water (moisture) is the sine qua non (that without which nothing else is valid) of skin health and a youthful firm complexion. Moisture is constantly evaporating from your skin, and also from the cosmetics that you buy or prepare. To keep the cosmetics spreadable and helpful to skin, humectants are added. A humectant is sometimes referred to as a hydrophilic substance, and it is just that: *hydro* means water and *philia* means love; humectants actually attract moisture from the air. Glycerin is such a substance; so is urea. One of the best natural hydrophilics is honey. If a humectant were not added to most creams, they would soon become dry and caked, and you wouldn't be able to spread them.

Skin-care products and cosmetics are designed to be used on the surface of your skin. To make them easy to apply they should be smooth, pleasant to touch, and thick enough to stay where they are applied. This requires chemical bulkers such as cellulose.

Colorants, flavorings, and fragrances are also part of every cosmetic or skin-care product. The more attractive a product is, the more often you'll use it. The more something is used, the greater the opportunity for it to effect change. Most creams and other cosmetics need at least two weeks to show results.

Here is a list of products that appear on the labels of cosmetics and also definitions of some of the terms that are essential to the discussion of cosmetics.

Acetic acid	Found in apples, grapes, oranges, pineapples, and other plants and fruits. A small percentage of vinegar is acetic acid. It stops bleeding and tones skin.
Acetone	The solvent in nail-polish remover.
Alcohol	Used in many cosmetics as a solvent.
Alkali	A caustic substance with a pH greater than 7. Sodium bicarbonate is an example of an alkali.
Allantoin	Used in creams and lotions for its calming and soothing effect. It is thought to encourage the growth of healthy tissue.
Almond meal	Pulverized almond meats.
Aloe vera	The sap or juice of the aloe plant. It is often used in cosmetics, but there is little scientific evidence that it actually promotes healing.
Alum	A product that is astringent and stops bleeding.
Ammonia	A strong alkaline product; mixed with peroxide, it bleaches hair.

Apricot	The crushed hulls make an excellent exfoliant. The oil is clear and soothing. The pulp of the fresh fruit can be used as a mask to soften the skin.
Astringent	A mixture of alcohol and other evaporative agents to make the skin feel tighter, smoother, and refreshed. Not for dry skin.
Azulene	An intensely blue liquid hydrocarbon (gasoline is a mixture of hydrocarbons) contained in the essential oil distilled from chamomile flowers. Small quantities are added to shampoos and other products to impart the characteristic odor of chamomile. Also used as a coloring agent. Reportedly an antiinflammatory agent. Nontoxic.
Baby oil	A mixture of mineral oil and vegetable oils. Can be used as a solvent for makeup, but many skin-care experts believe it actually has a drying effect on the skin.
Banana	A fruit high in potassium and pectin, makes a good dry-skin mask when mixed with oil.
Barrier	A heavy cream or lotion that protects the skin against evaporation. Any product that coats the skin can form a barrier. The most common is petroleum jelly.
Bath oil	Any oil added to your bath. You can make your own bath oils by mixing a small quantity of vegetable oil and a few drops of perfume together. It will float on the surface of the water and cling to your body, trapping moisture next to your skin.
Beer	The sugar and protein in beer thickens the hair if you use it as a setting lotion.
Bleach	Any product used for evening skin color, or for removing freckles or chloasma, is usually classified as a bleach.
Borax	A mild alkali that is used in laundry and in cleansing products.

Boric acid	An antiseptic powder that prevents bacterial growth.
Bracer	A skin bracer is essentially the same as a skin freshener. It usually has a high alcohol content and cools and refreshes the skin. Used as a term in men's cosmetics.
Buttermilk	The substance left after butter has been churned. It can also be made by adding cultures to milk, similar to the way yogurt is made. An excellent ingredient for the liquid part of facial masks.
Calamine	A combination of zinc oxide and iron oxide makes a pinkish powder used in lotions and ointments. It is astringent and very drying to the skin.
Calcium silicate	An anticaking agent that keeps powder dry, it absorbs water easily.
Camphor	A natural or synthetic substance that is also a moth repellent; it is included in skin fresheners to provide a cooling sensation.
Carotene	The yellow coloring from carrots and egg yolks, used as a coloring in cosmetics.
Castor oil	Used in cosmetics, especially eye oils and creams. It forms a tough, shiny film when it dries. Continued use is thought to encourage the growth of eyelashes.
Cellulose	A thickening agent used as an emulsifier in cosmetics.
Chalk	It is used as an alkali to reduce acidity, and is found in many antacids. It is also in tooth polishers and other products.
Chamomile	Used in teas or as the herbs in a sauna; can calm and clear the skin. The powdered flowers are used in many folklore recipes.
Cholesterol	Occurring in all animal fats and oils, it is used as an emulsifier and lubricant in cosmetics.

Cleansers

Lotions and creams used to clean the skin are called cleansers. These are used instead of soap, and are quite similar to each other.

Soap is in most of these products, but they also contain mineral oil, alcohol, water, and sometimes detergent. Most of these cleansers are designed to be tissued or rinsed off. If an oily surface is left on the face, a toner or astringent must be used to get the residue off. The toners or astringents almost always contain alcohol or another harsh solvent that removes the skin's surface oils as well as the cleanser.

Liquifying cleansing creams, designed to melt at body temperature, are similar to other cleansers. Washable creams are water soluble, and similar to soap, but are not suitable for oily skins. Milky cleansers are better for oily skins but also contain soap.

The scrubbing cleansers are usually just soft soaps with tiny grains that act as abrasives on the skin. It would be just as practical to dip a damp bar of a mild soap in salt or meal, and use that to abrade or wash the face.

Cocoa butter

Mae West used it as her basic beauty preparation, and it is an excellent skin softener and lubricant. It is a classic for pregnant women and seems to help avoid stretch marks.

Cod-liver oil

A pale yellow oil with a fishy odor used in creams and cosmetics. It contains vitamins A and D which promote healing. Can be used directly on the skin.

Cold cream

The original cream dates back to Greek times, and was probably a combination of olive oil and beeswax. It is solid at room temperature and liquifies on the skin. Some water is part of the formula; the evaporation of that water causes the cooling effect.

Collagen

A protein substance found in the connective tissue of all animals. It is the breakdown of the collagen fibers in skin that contributes to the formation of wrinkles. Collagen is not absorbed by the skin, and a collagen cream, although pleasant and protective, does not affect the skin's structure or condition.

Cornmeal	A grain that is used in exfoliating the upper layer of skin.
Cornstarch	Used in powders and depilatories, it absorbs water and is soothing to the skin.
Cucumber	Slices can be used as an astringent mask.
Dandruff	A condition of the scalp usually caused by excessive dryness or excessive oiliness. Many of the popular dandruff shampoos actually exfoliate the skin of the scalp to get rid of the excess scales. After the exfoliation—often with the use of salicylic acid or resorcinol—the hair is washed. Sulfur and tar are also used to cut down on the scaling by slowing cell growth.
Dentifrice	A paste or powder used with a brush to clean the teeth. It usually contains an amazing array of ingredients, including a number of abrasives and flavors.
Deodorants	A combination of aluminum chloride, urea, and other substances that control the odor caused by the action of bacteria on perspiration. A deodorant does not stop the perspiration; it cuts down on the bacteria action, and perfumes in the products mask the smell of the bacteria.
Depilatory	A chemical method of ridding the skin of unwanted hair, these usually contain hydrogen sulfide. They act by dissolving the hair and can be very drying and irritating to the skin. Never leave the depilatory on longer than the suggested time on the directions that come with the product.
Detergent	A group of synthetic cleansers that can be used in hard water. Detergents do not leave a hard water scum, and many of them have a wetting agent that helps them to work quickly. Usually they are alkaline, but in cosmetic products they can have a pH balance close to that of normal skin.

Egg	Dehydrated egg powder is often included in cosmetics and shampoos on the theory that it will provide protein that is beneficial. The oil of the egg yolk mixes easily with other oils and is used as a basis for masks and cosmetics. Be sure you keep your egg facial cool; it can become sticky and hard if you attempt to wash it away with hot water.
Elder flowers	Used as a tea and in skin and eye lotions, it is mildly astringent and keeps the skin soft and clean. Slightly diuretic, it can help to control water retention.
Emollient	Creams, lotions, moisturizers, and softeners are all emollients. There is little difference among them except for the amount of water they contain. These preparations are all aimed at making the skin feel softer and retarding fine wrinkles. If an emollient has a low melting point, it will feel greasy; with a high melting point it will soak quickly into the skin. Most are colorless. Petroleum jelly is considered an emollient with a low melting point.
Emulsifiers	These are agents such as potassium that will keep fats suspended in water, resulting in a thick liquid that looks milky. Emulsifiers are needed to prevent oil and water from separating in creams and lotions.
Estrogen	A female hormone.
Ether	A compound that is not soluble in either water or oil, it is used in nail-polish removers and in the polish itself. Avoid inhaling ether; it can make you dizzy.
Eucalyptus oil	A pale yellow liquid that comes from the fresh leaves of the eucalyptus tree. It smells a bit like camphor and can be used as an antiseptic.
Eye oils	Special eye creams are usually emulsions that have a high percentage of oils. Eye oils or creams usually contain no perfume.

Eye pencils and eyeliners	A tiny thin line drawn around the eye accentuates its form. The technique is used to make eyes look larger. Most of the waterproof liners must be removed with an oil, and it is the removal of the eyeliner that causes as much irritation as anything else. George Masters, a Hollywood makeup artist, advises his clients not to use shadow or liner because applying and removing it tend to stretch the delicate skin.
Eye shadow	Usually in shades of blue, green, brown, or gray, eye shadow comes in cream or powder form. More problems of itching, burning, and swelling result from eye makeup and mascara than from any other cosmetic.
Eyedrops and washes	These are designed to soothe and clear the redness in the eyes. To contract red blood vessels tetrahydrozoline is used. Be sure that the bottle you have is kept as clean as possible.
Eyelash creams and oils	Designed to make the lashes soft and shiny, they often are the cause of allergic reactions. Castor oil and peach-kernel oil are two of the popular oils used in these products.
Facial pack	This is just an old-fashioned name for facial mask. They are designed to do one of two things: either to tighten pores and stimulate or to remove wrinkles and relax. The tightening and cooling sensations in some masks are brought about by evaporation. The warming and nourishing benefits are probably brought about by preventing evaporation, through the use of oils.
Fennel	Used in astringents and perfumes, this is an herb. A compress of fennel tea can soothe irritated eyes, but may cause an allergic reaction.
Folic acid	A vitamin of the B-complex group and an important nutrient for skin health.
Foundation	The basic skin-covering makeup. Some contain as much as 75 percent water; others are available in a hard, dry stick with a very low percentage of water. Generally the harder the product, the more opaque the covering.

Freckle	A dark spot on the skin; lentigines, or age spots in anyone over 30.
Freshener	A weak astringent, usually a clear liquid, designed to make the skin feel tight and cool. It is about 60 percent witch hazel and usually about 15 percent camphorated alcohol and 1 percent citric acid. It can also contain other ingredients or perfumes.
Fuller's earth	A variety of kaolin, which is a fine clay. Used in the treatment of oily skin, it absorbs fats and oils on the surface of the skin. It also absorbs water and can be drying.
Gel	A clear semisolid that is jellylike. Lip glosses are gels that protect the lips by forming a barrier between the lips and the air. They do not carry as much color as a lipstick.
Gelatin	Used in cosmetics and especially hair-setting and nail products. You can create a gelatin mask by just applying slightly warm gelatin to the face and allowing it to harden. The mask will protect the skin from evaporation, and pick up dead, loose cells.
Ginseng	A popular oriental plant root that has the reputation of soothing and healing properties.
Glucose	Used as a skin soother. It occurs naturally in blood and grapes, and in corn it is a natural sweetener.
Glycerin	A solvent and humectant, it helps keep the moisture in creams and other products by attracting moisture from the surrounding atmosphere. It is a basic ingredient in many masks and hand lotions. Glycerin and rose water make an excellent hand softener, but cannot improve the condition of the skin.
Grapefruit oil	Oil from the outer surface of the grapefruit skin.
Grape-seed oil	A very fine oil that is used in watchmaking and also in cosmetics.

Gum	Water-soluble thickeners that can be either natural or synthetic are used in all sorts of cosmetics.
Gum tragacanth	An emulsifier that is used in everything from creams and toothpaste to rouges and hand lotions; it is a plant product.
Henna	This ancient cosmetic was used for dyeing the hair and also the palms and soles of the feet. Its advantage is that very few people are allergic to henna, but it should not be used for dyeing eyelashes or eyebrows.
Hexachlorophene	An antibacterial that was restricted by the government over a dozen years ago, hexachlorophene is toxic in concentrated doses.
Honey	A sweet, syrupy material made by bees. It attracts moisture from the air, and has been used in cosmetics since the days of early Egypt.
Hormones	Used in creams and lotions; estrogen or protesterone are often added to help thicken aging skin. The benefits are uncertain, but they do make the creams much more expensive because the hormones themselves are expensive.
Humectant	A substance that attracts moisture from the air or from the surrounding atmosphere; usually found in creams and lotions.
Hydrocarbons	Petroleum, natural gas, coal, and charcoal are all hydrocarbons. They can be used to keep water from evaporating.
Hydroquinone	A white phenol used in bleach and freckle creams and in some suntan preparations. If you leave the cover off a cream containing hydroquinone, the cream will turn brown in a short time.
Hypoallergenic	The term used for a substance that is free of allergens. There really is no such product, however, because someone, somewhere, is allergic to everything.

Iodine	A trace element important to the action of the thyroid and the rate of metabolism. It is associated with acne and most doctors suggest a low-iodine diet to avoid eruptions.
Ivy extract	Taken from the evergreen leaves of a European plant, it is used in tightening the skin of the body and face. Many cellulite preparations depend on ivy extract for their "firming" action.
Japan wax	A pale yellow fat used as a substitute for beeswax in cosmetics.
Jasmine	Oil of a climbing plant with a white flower, this is used to scent cosmetics.
Kaolin	A white clay powder used in cosmetic masks and taken for stomach troubles. Originally found in China, it is now found in Europe.
Keratin	A protein substance from the horns, hooves and hair of animals. It is part of our outer skin and nails as well.
Ketones	The solvents used in nail polish and nail-polish removers. It is also known by the name acetone.
Lactic acid	Used in skin fresheners, it is mildly exfoliating and makes the skin look fresher and newer. It is found in milk, beer, sauerkraut, pickles, and yogurt as well as in other foods made by fermentation.
Lactose	A milk sugar often used as the basis for skin lotions and hand creams. You can make your own cream by mixing lactose powder with oil.
Lanolin	The oil glands of a sheep are similar to those of a human, and the oil from these glands is probably closer than any other to the natural human-skin oils. Lanolin is used in almost all cosmetics and in hair conditioners, lotions, and creams. Lanolin contains about 30 percent water, and without that water it would be quite waxy. It often causes allergies.

Lard	The fat from the hog. Lard is an excellent emollient and the base of many soaps and creams. It is insoluble in water and is a good barrier cream. Pork fat has been used to rub away blackheads in folk-remedy formulas.
Lead	Avoid any cosmetic with lead because it can cause a myriad of unpleasant toxic effects.
Lecithin	A natural antioxidant, found in oil-tempera and other paints; in cosmetics it is used in creams, lipsticks, lotions and soaps. A natural emulsifier and spreading agent, it is insoluble in water, but swells when immersed.
Lemon	The most popular of all the fruits used in cosmetics. It is about 7 percent citric acid and is often used as a hair rinse to rid the hair of any alkaline soap scum. Lemon should be diluted with water if it is used for a bleach on the face or hands.
Lemon oil	The slightly oily solution that comes from squeezing the skin of the fruit.
Lime	A small citrus fruit with a very acid pulp and juice. Used as a flavoring. Lime juice can turn the skin brown when used as a hand cream or cleanser.
Lime water	A water solution of calcium hydroxide that absorbs carbon dioxide from the air. *Not* the juice of the lime.
Linoleic acid	A fatty acid prepared from edible fats and oils.
Lipstick	A mixture of wax and red or orange pigments. The formulas vary from manufacturer to manufacturer. Most formulas contain a small amount of castor oil, dyes, and lanolin. In most lipsticks the largest ingredient is beeswax. Swollen, cracked, or very dry lips might indicate you are having an adverse reaction to your lipstick. Herpes can be transmitted through sharing lipsticks; don't use "tester" lipsticks at cosmetic counters.

Liquifying cream	This is another term for a cleansing cream that liquifies on the face. It is very much like cold cream and contains mineral oil, water, and borax.
Lovage	An aromatic herb that has deodorant properties.
Magnesia	A skin freshener and powder that is an excellent mask for oily skins when mixed with water to form a paste.
Mallow	An herb that is used for red and purple coloring.
Mascara	A coloring for the eyelashes. It contains insoluble ingredients, such as paraffin and lanolin. The black color comes from iron oxides and carbon. Some mascaras include fibers of nylon or rayon that thicken and extend the lashes; they are glued to the lashes with thick mascara. Mascara should never be shared. Cake mascara gives some of the best control.
Matte makeup	An all-in-one makeup that is color and powder in a tube or cake. It has excellent coverage, but makes wrinkled skin look more wrinkled.
Mayonnaise	A soft, light salad dressing that has all the ingredients which are naturally soothing to the skin: oil, egg yolk, and vinegar. It is an excellent body, neck, and facial mask. To improve skin texture, apply mayonnaise and then wrap a warm, moist towel around the treated part of your body.
Medicated makeup	Usually used for oily, blemished skins, it contains antibacterial agents and is very drying.
Menthol	A mild anesthetic, it gives a cool feeling to the skin and is obtained from peppermint or other mint oils.
Mica	A group of minerals found in crystalline form. They provide color in eye shadows and other makeups, and are responsible for the shimmer or pearlized effect in cosmetics.
Milk	Used in cosmetics and for bath products. It is soothing for the skin, but it must be rinsed from the skin carefully because it sours and turns rancid easily.

Mineral oil	An oil used in infant and adult creams. When heated it smells like petroleum, from which it is derived. It is a lubricant, protective, and binding oil, and it is popular because it has an indefinite shelf life and needs no refrigeration.
Mink oil	The oils from the skin of the mink, thought by some to have special softening properties, but none have been proven.
Mint	Used in astringents and oils, it is tingling and refreshing.
Mordant	A chemical used to fix a dye. Used in hair colorants.
Mouthwash	The basic mouthwash is an alkaline that contains alcohol, water, and flavorings as well as some sodium bicarbonate. They mask the odor of bacteria at work in the mouth.
Mucilage	A solution of vegetable or animal gums and water. Used as a soother in skin masks.
Mud Packs	A mask that contains "mud," usually in the form of a high grade of clay.
Musk	A smelly substance taken from the glands of the Asian deer which leaves this substance on trees and foliage to attract the female deer. It is a very attractive scent to some people.
Myristic acid	Used in soaps, cleansers, and shampoos, it is a natural substance that comes from butter acids. It is used to make soap lather easily.
Nail bleaches	Compounds to get ink and other stains off the fingers. Bleaches usually include titanium, zinc, and petroleum jelly as well as mineral oil and some perfume.
Nail enamel (polish)	A mixture of chemicals and pigments that coats the nails with color.
Nail hardeners	A protective, polishlike coating for the nails that contains formaldehyde or silicone.

Nail-polish removers	Most contain a large percentage of acetone and are very drying to the nail.
Niacinamide	A B vitamin used as a skin stimulant, it is a white or yellow crystalline powder. Taking large amounts can bring on a flush and stimulate the blood supply.
Note	A term used to identify a smell or taste in the perfume business.
Oatmeal	Popular as a skin-soother and face mask. It is especially good for removing dirt from sensitive skins and can be used instead of soap.
Oleic acid	An oily acid that has excellent skin-penetrating properties. Used in foundations and shaving preparations.
Olive oil	The reason why so many Mediterranean people have good skin. Superior to mineral oils in its ability to penetrate the skin, it is a popular massage oil and scalp treatment. Also an excellent food oil.
Opacifier	Fatty alcohols or other substances to create a makeup impervious to light. Some concealers use these opacifying agents to help block out discolorations and blemishes.
Orange oil	A liquid squeezed from the peel of a fresh ripe orange. Many people are allergic to this, but it is used to scent perfumes and soaps.
Oxalic acid	Used in freckle and skin bleaches, it is a caustic substance and may cause irritation of the mucous membranes.
Palm-kernel oil	An edible yellow oil often used in salad dressings, it is also used in soaps, baby products, and lubricants.
Papaya	A fruit grown in tropical countries. The meat is pinky-orange and very sweet. The fruit and rind contain an enzyme used as a meat tenderizer because it can dissolve dead material. It is used in skin peelers and is very potent.

Paraffin	A distilled waxy substance that comes from petroleum. It melts easily and is used to form an air-tight seal when preserving fruits and vegetables at home. Once used in breast implants, it has caused cancer in mice. There is no problem known when used on the surface of the skin. It is the thickener used in lipsticks, creams, and so on. Usually one of the ingredients in mascara.
Peanut oil	A vegetable oil that is also used in the manufacture of soaps, hair-grooming aids, creams, and ointments. It can be greenish in color, and is often combined with olive oil or almond oil because it is less expensive and can be used as an extender.
Pectin	An emulsifier used in place of gums. Pectin is found in bananas and apples, and is considered a thickening agent as well as a stomach soother.
Peppermint oil	Used in toilet waters, fresheners, and toothpaste. It is mildly anaesthetic and can be used as a healing cleanser.
Perfume	A combination of herbal and floral oils that provides an attractive fragrance when applied to the skin.
Peroxide	A bleach that can affect hair and skin. It is irritating and even injurious to the eyes.
Petrolatum	Another name for petroleum jelly. It is used in many cosmetics and creams and emollients. A good lubricant, it gives lipstick or gloss its shine, and it also softens and smooths skin by coating it with an oily film that prevents evaporation.
pH	A scale used to measure the alkaline/acid balance of a substance. Water is thought to be neutral at 7 in the scale of 0 to 14, with 0 the most acid and 14 the most alkaline. The skin is usually about 5 pH, slightly acidic.
Phenol	Another term for carbolic acid. It is an anaesthetic, but it can also cause burns and peeling. Swallowing even a small amount can cause nausea, vomiting, and convulsions. Fatal poisoning can also occur through skin absorption. It is used in chemical skin peels under the direction of a doctor. It should be handled with care and caution.

Photosensitivity | Sensitivity to certain chemicals that cause darkening of the skin when it is exposed to sunlight. Figs are a photosensitive substance; some perfumes, celery, vanilla, bergamot, some anti-bacteria soaps, bromides, and tetracycline in medicine can also cause skin to darken.

Pine tar | A thick, blackish liquid used in dandruff shampoos. It is slightly irritating to skin, and causes mild peeling.

Pineapple juice | The juice of the pineapple, it has protein-digesting properties similar to that of the papaya.

Placenta | Prepared from the placenta (the lining of the womb that is expelled after birth), it is rich in nutrients, and used by cosmetic manufacturers as the basis of some skin creams.

Pomade | A hair cream or dressing, usually thick and waxy. It makes the hair shiny and stiff.

Potassium Carbonate | Odorless powder used in bleaching creams and some cosmetic creams. It has a peeling action, and is potentially irritating.

Powder | A fine, dusty substance applied to the face or body. It gives the skin a velvety finish and subdues any shine. Most face powders are talc, kaolin, zinc oxide, and other materials such as corn or rice starch, or even potato starch. The color of the powder is provided by pigments, and changes according to fashion.

Preservative | A substance that retards decay. Most cosmetics must include preservatives or they would have a very short shelf-life.

Progesterone | A female sex hormone used in cosmetics. Like estrogen, it is often included in cosmetics to retard wrinkling, but there is no evidence that it works.

Proteins | The essential substance of living cells, a complex of oxygen, nitrogen, carbon, and hydrogen. Cosmetic manufacturers create formulas that protect the protein of the skin and hair. The surface of the skin and hair is mostly protein.

Pumice	An abrasive stone ground into skin-cleansing and thinning pastes and cleansers. It rubs away hair and calluses on the surface of the skin. Too much rubbing can be irritating.
Resorcinol	A peeling agent that is antiseptic and astringent. It can cause allergic reactions. Resorcinol is included in many acne preparations. Very drying to the skin.
Rhubarb	A plant with edible stalks and poisonous leaves. The juice can be used as a hair tint for blond shades.
Rice starch	A fine powder included in face and body powders.
Rosin	A yellow, sticky substance that comes from pine trees; it is used in depilatories and soaps.
Rouge	A powdery red colorant used to tint the cheeks. Cakes include kaolin and coloring matter. A higher percentage of powder and the rouge is a blusher; a higher percentage of wax and it is a paste. Some rouges come in cream form, but they are not recommended because they clog the pores.
Royal jelly	The secretion of the honeybee, it is a mixture of fats and proteins. It has been touted as an antiwrinkle ingredient, but there is no evidence that it works.
Safflower oil	A vegetable oil used in cooking, it is very vulnerable to exposure to the air. Used in creams and lotions, it is similar to sesame oil and will soften the skin.
Salicylic acid	One of the main ingredients in aspirin, it has a peeling and exfoliating effect on the skin. It occurs naturally in wintergreen and birch, and those plants have been used for medicinal teas. It is often in acne and skin-renewal preparations.
Sesame oil	A food vegetable oil that can also be used for grooming and cosmetics. Often used in sunscreen preparations and massage creams. It is similar in texture to olive oil.
Setting lotions	A formula of water and gums that keeps the hair in place. It usually can be used as a skin mask as well.

Shampoo

Packaged in tubes and bottles, these hair cleansers are usually about 25 percent soap and about 50 percent water and oils.

Shark-liver oil

A rich source of vitamin A frequently used in hand cream.

Silica

A white powder that is a fine grade of sand used in powders and eye shadows. Silicas can also be used in exfoliants and cleansing masks.

Silicones

Fluid oils, resins, and compounds that can be formulated from silica. They are used in nail polishes and creams and lotions. They stick to the skin, and are seldom toxic.

Slippery elm bark

The sap of this tree is used in masks and skin tighteners.

Soap

The best of all cleansers; the development of soap about 1,000 years ago doubled the population of Europe by cutting down on infection. Soaps vary in content from a mild fatty acid soap to a strongly alkaline soap. The lower the pH, the milder the soap. Clear soaps such as Neutrogena are nonalkaline and include glycerin. Some soaps include antibacterial ingredients to combat surface bacteria and its odor.

You can make your own soap from vegetable oil and a caustic, such as lye, but it is far better to buy a soap that seems compatible with your skin. It is very important to rinse away any soap residue. Soap can be found in cleansers, toothpaste, shaving products, and even creams.

Sodium benzoate

A white antiseptic powder. It is used as a preservative in foods and in cosmetics to keep oily substances from becoming rancid.

Sodium
   bicarbonate

This is commonly used under the name of baking soda and is a skin-soothing white crystal. It is a gentle alkaline wash that can neutralize an acid. A mixture of vegetable oil, sodium bicarbonate, and a little vinegar makes an excellent skin cleanser.

Sodium carbonate	These small, odorless crystals absorb water from the air and are used in bath salts and soaps. Toxic when swallowed.
Sodium hydroxide	The common name is soda lye; it is an alkaline emulsifier used in food preparation and also one of the ingredients in most soaps, shampoos, and shaving soaps.
Sorbic acid	A powder made from berries, it is included in creams as a binder. It is used in cosmetics as a preservative and as a substitute for glycerin.
Sorbitol	A replacement for glycerin.
Soybean oil	A yellow oil used mainly in margarine. It can clog pores.
Spermaceti	Used as a base in creams and cleansers, it is a wax from the oil of the sperm whale. It is being replaced by jojoba oil.
Starch	Used in powders, colorings, shampoos, and bath salts, starch absorbs moisture. As a basic ingredient it is used in face powders because it imparts a velvet finish. Usually it is insoluble in cold water, but can be dissolved in boiling water.
Stearic acid	A white, waxy fatty acid, it is used in soaps and lubricants; most cosmetic creams contain this product. Used in deodorants, antiperspirants, foundations, and hand creams or lotions, it gives a pearly luminescence to the lotion.
Stiffener	An ingredient, usually a gum, used to add body to creams or soaps.
Styptic	Usually sold in the form of a stick or pencil, it is a combination of ingredients that contracts the blood vessels and stops bleeding.
Sugar	Used as a substitute for glycerin, it combines easily with water. In granulated form it can be used as an abrasive for the skin.

Sulfur

An antiseptic used to stimulate the scalp and to speed the drying of acne.

Sun-block cream

Usually a combination of mineral oil, lanolin, water, and sun blockers.

Talc

Finely powdered magnesium silicate, talc gives a smooth, slippery feel to face powders and to creams. It is one of the ingredients in rouges, face masks, and foot-drying preparations.

Tallow

Thick, waxy fat from animals. It is used in lipsticks and soaps.

Tannic acid

A mild astringent used in sun preparations. Tea contains tannic acid and tea-bag compresses seem to soothe and tighten the skin's pores.

Texturizer

Any chemical that improves the texture of a lotion or cream by making it smooth and creamy.

Thyme

An herb used as a flavoring for mouthwashes and shaving lotions.

Toilet water

A mixture of alcohol and perfume oils that produces a weak perfumed water which is refreshing but very drying.

Turtle oil

An oil from the bodies of turtles that is touted as being helpful in the elimination of wrinkles.

Umber

A brown earth that is used in powders and eye shadows.

Urea

A product excreted in human and animal urine. It is a hydrophilac and antiseptic.

Vegetable gums and oils

Vegetable by-products used in cosmetics. The advantage is that very few have any known toxicity.

Vinegar

Used to remove alkaline scum or residue after washing the face or hair, it is a solvent for cosmetic oils and resins, containing a very low percentage of acetic acid. Spraying the face with a solution of apple cider vinegar and water often preserves the acidic surface of the skin and keeps it blemish-free.

Vitamins	Found in varying proportions in most foods or organic compounds, vitamins are essential for regulating normal growth and functioning of the skin. Each vitamin plays a specific role in maintaining the processes of life, and no vitamin is able to substitute for another.
Water	The major ingredient in all living matter, it is the most popular ingredient in foods, cosmetics, and drugs.
Wax	Oily substance obtained from plants and animals.
Wheat germ	A popular food also used in cosmetic masks. Contains a high percentage of vitamin E.
Wheat gluten	Used in powders and creams as a thickener.
Witch hazel	A skin freshener made from the leaves and twigs of a plant. It is an anesthetic and astringent that also has a low tannic acid content.
Xylene	A colorless liquid made from coal tar and gas. It is a degreaser and is used in the removal of lacquers and nail polishes.
Yucca	A plant of the Southwest used in the making of organic cosmetics.
Zinc oxide	A creamy white ointment used to protect the skin. Used in skin bleaches, face masks, and antiperspirants, zinc oxide is probably the most basic of all skin ointments. It is astringent, antiseptic, and protects against sunburn.

Index

℗

PLUME Titles for a Better Life